HIGH PROTEIN COOKBOOK FOR WOMEN

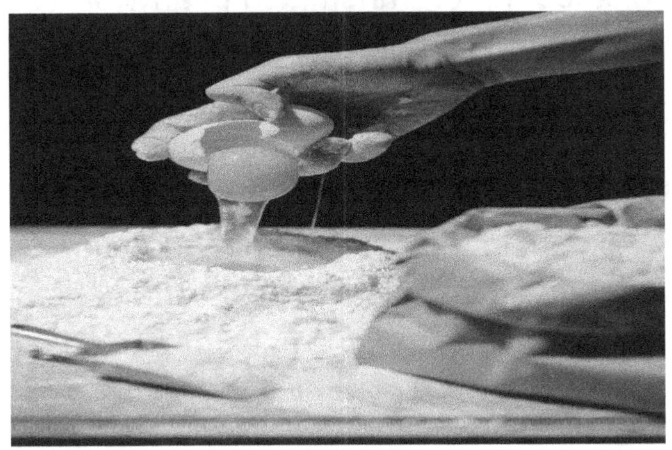

"Empowering Women Through Nourishment: A High Protein Culinary Odyssey for Strength, Vitality, and Well-Being"

EMMA LYNCH

TABLE OF CONTENTS

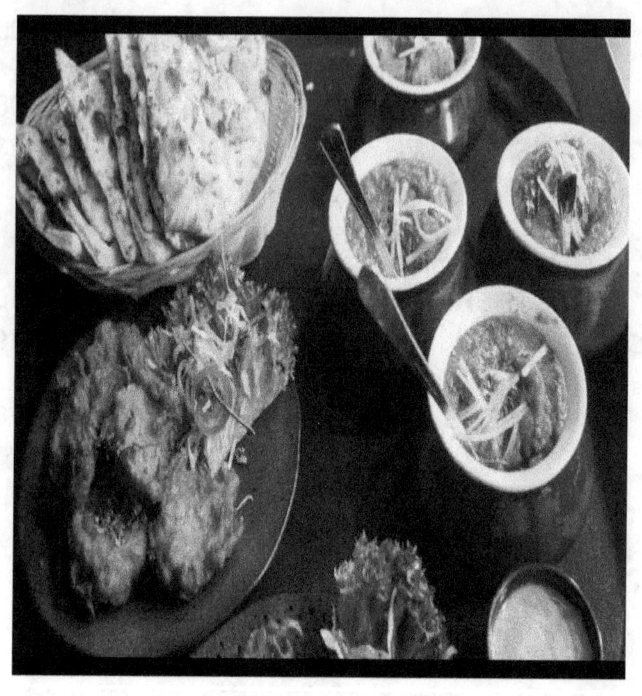

INTRODUCTION

Welcome to the "High Protein Cookbook for Women," a culinary journey crafted to empower and nourish the incredible strength and vitality of women. In a world where health and well-being take center stage, the importance of a balanced and protein-rich diet cannot be overstated. This cookbook is designed to be your trusted companion on this transformative quest towards a healthier and more vibrant you.

As women, our bodies undergo unique changes and challenges throughout life, from adolescence to motherhood and beyond. The role of nutrition in supporting these dynamic phases is pivotal. Protein, often hailed as the building block of life, plays a crucial role in muscle repair, energy metabolism, and overall cellular function. Yet, finding delicious and diverse ways to incorporate ample protein into our diets can sometimes be a culinary puzzle.

This cookbook is not just a collection of recipes; it's a comprehensive guide tailored to meet the specific nutritional needs of women. Whether you're an active fitness enthusiast, a busy professional, or someone seeking to enhance your overall well-being, these recipes are crafted with you in mind. From breakfast to dinner, and every snack in between, each dish is a celebration of flavor, nutrition, and the joy of wholesome eating.

Before delving into the tantalizing recipes that await you, take a moment to explore the foundational chapters. Learn why protein is essential for women, discover how to set personalized protein goals, and gain insights into the art of mindful eating and portion control. Whether you're new to the kitchen or a seasoned chef, the cooking tips and meal planning strategies provided will guide you on a seamless and enjoyable culinary adventure.

Embrace the journey of nourishing your body with foods that not only satisfy your taste buds but also fortify your strength and resilience. Here's to a cookbook that goes beyond recipes, inviting you to cultivate a lifestyle that supports your health and empowers your journey as a woman. Get ready to embark on a flavorful odyssey where each dish is a step towards a stronger, healthier, and more vibrant you. Cheers to the art of high-protein living!

CHAPTER ONE

UNDERSTANDING THE IMPORTANCE OF PROTEIN FOR WOMEN

In the realm of women's health and wellness, the role of protein extends far beyond mere sustenance. Delve into the multifaceted significance of protein, recognizing it as a pivotal component for holistic well-being:

1. **Muscle Health and Tone:
   - Protein is essential for maintaining and growing lean muscular mass. For women, this is particularly significant, contributing to overall strength, tone, and a healthy physique. Adequate protein intake supports muscle repair and growth, fostering a sculpted and resilient body.

2. Hormonal Harmony:
   - Hormonal balance is vital for women's health, influencing various aspects of well-being, including mood, energy levels, and reproductive health. Protein is instrumental in supporting the synthesis of hormones, contributing to a harmonious and balanced endocrine system.

3. Metabolic Boost and Weight Management:

- Protein-rich foods have a higher thermic effect, meaning they require more energy for digestion and absorption. This metabolic boost can aid in weight management by enhancing calorie expenditure and promoting a feeling of fullness, which can be particularly beneficial for women striving to maintain a healthy weight.

4. Energy and Vitality:
- Protein serves as a sustained source of energy, providing a stable and long-lasting fuel source. This is especially valuable for women with active lifestyles, helping to sustain energy levels throughout the day and supporting optimal physical performance.

5. Immune System Support:
- The immune system relies on protein to produce antibodies and enzymes that help combat infections and illnesses. A sufficient intake of protein contributes to a robust immune system, enhancing a woman's ability to fend off common ailments and maintain overall health.

6. Collagen Production for Skin Health:
- Collagen, a protein abundant in the skin, provides structural support and elasticity. Adequate protein intake supports collagen production, contributing to skin health, suppleness, and a youthful complexion—an aspect of particular interest to many women.

7. Reproductive Health:
   - Protein is integral for reproductive health, supporting the development and maintenance of tissues crucial for fertility and pregnancy. Adequate protein is vital during various life stages, including puberty, pregnancy, and menopause.

8. Cognitive Function and Mood Regulation:
   - Proteins are the building blocks of neurotransmitters, the chemical messengers that play a role in mood regulation and cognitive function. Ensuring an ample supply of protein supports mental well-being, concentration, and emotional stability.

9. Hair and Nail Strength:
   - Keratin, a structural protein, contributes to the strength and health of hair and nails. Adequate protein intake promotes the production of keratin, enhancing the resilience and aesthetics of these external features.

10. Optimal Recovery and Resilience:
   - For women engaged in physical activities, protein is instrumental in post-exercise recovery. It aids in muscle repair, reduces soreness, and enhances overall resilience, allowing women to pursue their fitness goals with vigor.

Understanding the multifaceted importance of protein for women goes beyond the conventional view of a nutrient. It is a dynamic and integral aspect of women's health, supporting various physiological functions that contribute to strength, vitality, and overall well-being. Whether through lean meats, plant-based sources, or a combination of both, prioritizing protein is a cornerstone of a holistic approach to women's health.

CHAPTER TWO

SETTING UP YOUR KITCHEN

Creating a kitchen tailored for protein-packed cooking involves thoughtful consideration of both tools and ingredients. Here's a comprehensive guide on setting up your kitchen for a successful high-protein culinary adventure:

Essential Tools for Protein-Packed Cooking

1. **Quality Knives:**
   - Sharp knives are indispensable for precise cutting of various protein sources. Invest in a set of quality knives for tasks ranging from trimming meats to finely chopping vegetables.

2. **Cutting Boards:**
   - To prevent cross-contamination, have separate cutting boards for different protein types – one for meat, one for poultry, and another for fish. This ensures food safety and preserves distinct flavors.

3. **Cookware Assortment:**
   - A well-rounded set of cookware is essential. Pots, pans, and baking sheets cater to various cooking methods like grilling, baking, sautéing, and

simmering, allowing you to diversify your protein-centric recipes.

4. **Digital Food Scale:**
   - Precision in portion control is key, especially when managing protein intake. A digital food scale enables accurate measurements, aiding adherence to dietary guidelines and achieving nutritional goals.

5. **Blender or Food Processor:**
   - These versatile appliances open doors to a range of protein-packed culinary creations. Blenders are perfect for smoothies and shakes, while food processors assist in chopping, blending, and creating flavorful sauces or spreads.

6. **Grill or Grill Pan:**
   - Enhance the taste and texture of proteins by incorporating grilling into your repertoire. Whether using an outdoor grill or a stovetop grill pan, this tool adds a delightful char and depth of flavor to lean meats and vegetables.

7. **Instant-Read Thermometer:**
   - Ensure your proteins are perfectly cooked by investing in an instant-read thermometer. This tool takes the guesswork out of cooking, providing accurate readings for safe and delicious results.

8. **Storage Containers:**
   - Streamline meal prep and storage with a variety of containers. They facilitate organized storage of

prepped ingredients and leftovers, supporting a systematic and efficient approach to your high-protein lifestyle.

Must-Have Ingredients for Success

1. **Lean Protein Sources:**
   - Stock up on lean meats such as chicken, turkey, fish, and lean cuts of beef or pork. These form the foundation of protein-packed meals.

2. **Plant-Based Proteins:**
   - Diversify your protein sources with plant-based options like tofu, tempeh, legumes, and quinoa. These provide essential nutrients for both vegetarians and those looking to vary their protein intake.

3. **Eggs:**
   - Eggs are an affordable and adaptable source of protein. They can be incorporated into various dishes, from breakfast omelets to baked goods.

4. **Greek Yogurt:**
   - Rich in protein and probiotics, Greek yogurt is a versatile ingredient suitable for both sweet and savory recipes.

5. **Nuts and Seeds:**

   - Add texture, flavor, and healthy fats to your
meals with a variety of nuts and seeds. They are
excellent for salads, snacks, and even as toppings
for yogurt.

6. **Whole Grains:**
   - Incorporate whole grains like brown rice, quinoa,
and oats for a well-rounded and fiber-rich diet.
These grains complement proteins, creating
satisfying and nutritious meals.

7. **Herbs and Spices:**
   - Elevate the flavor of your dishes without relying
on excessive salt or unhealthy condiments. A
well-stocked spice rack allows you to experiment
and enhance the taste of your protein-packed
creations.

8. **Healthy Oils:**
   - Choose cooking oils such as olive oil or
avocado oil for healthier fats. These oils add
richness to your dishes while aligning with a
high-protein, nutritious lifestyle.

Setting up your kitchen with these essential tools
and ingredients lays the groundwork for a
successful and enjoyable protein-packed culinary
journey. Whether you're a seasoned chef or a
cooking novice, a well-equipped kitchen makes the
process smoother and more rewarding. So, gather
your tools, stock your pantry, and get ready to

savor the delicious benefits of a protein-rich lifestyle.

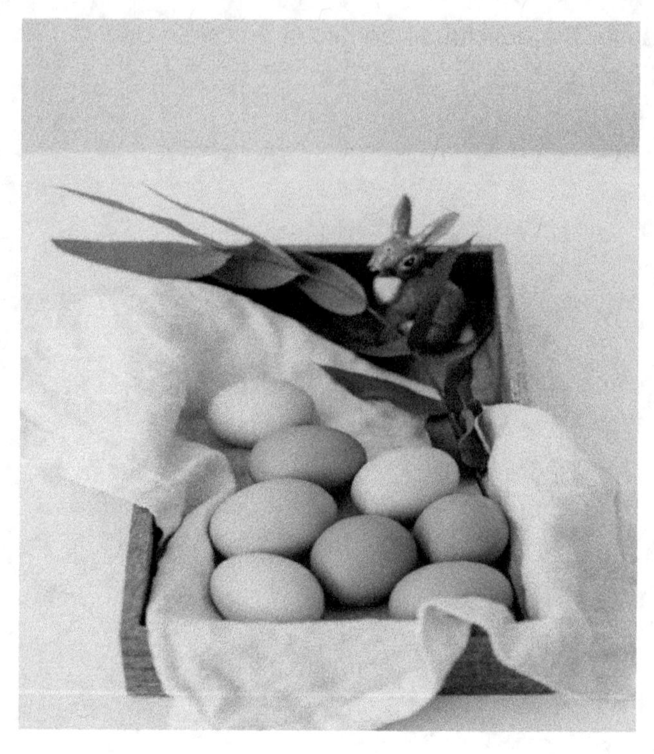

CHAPTER THREE

BREAKFAST BOOSTERS

"Breakfast Boosters" are energizing and nutritious elements you can add to your morning meal to kickstart your day. Here are some ideas to enhance your breakfast with nutritional benefits and sustained energy:

1. **Protein-Packed Start:**
   - Incorporate protein-rich foods like eggs, Greek yogurt, cottage cheese, or smoked salmon to keep you full and provide essential amino acids.

2. **Whole Grains:**
   - Choose whole grain options such as oatmeal, whole wheat toast, or quinoa for complex carbohydrates, fiber, and sustained energy.

3. **Healthy Fats:**
   - Avocado slices, chia seeds, or a sprinkle of nuts/seeds can add healthy fats, promoting satiety and supporting brain function.

4. **Fruits and Berries:**
   - Fresh fruits and berries not only add natural sweetness but also contribute vitamins, minerals, and antioxidants.

5. **Leafy Greens:**

- Sneak in some spinach or kale into a morning smoothie or omelet for an extra dose of vitamins and minerals.

6. **Smoothie Power:**
   - Blend a nutrient-packed smoothie with a combination of fruits, vegetables, protein powder, and a liquid of your choice (milk, yogurt, or a dairy-free alternative).

7. **Hydration:**
   - Drink a glass of water to rehydrate your body after a restful night's sleep.

8. **Caffeine Kick:**
   - If you enjoy coffee or tea, consider including it in your breakfast routine for a gentle caffeine boost.

Remember, a balanced breakfast sets a positive tone for the day, providing the energy and nutrients your body needs. Feel free to mix and match these "Breakfast Boosters" based on your preferences and dietary requirements.

PROTEIN-PACKED SMOOTHIE BOWLS

Creating a protein-packed smoothie bowl is a delicious and nutritious way to start your day. Here's a simple guide to crafting a satisfying protein-rich smoothie bowl:

Ingredients:

1. **Base:**
   - 1-1.5 cups of frozen fruits (e.g., berries, banana, mango)
   - 1/2 cup of Greek yogurt or plant-based yogurt for creaminess and added protein
   - 1/4 cup of liquid (milk, almond milk, or your preferred liquid)

2. **Protein Boosters:**
   - One scoop of collagen, plant-based, or whey protein powder of your choice
   - 1-2 tablespoons of nut butter (almond butter, peanut butter) for additional protein and richness

3. **Toppings:**
   - Chia seeds, flaxseeds, or hemp seeds for extra fiber and protein
   - Fresh fruit slices or berries for added vitamins and natural sweetness
   - Granola for complex carbs and crunch
   - Nuts or seeds (e.g., almonds, pumpkin seeds) for texture and healthy fats
   - Shredded coconut or cacao nibs for a flavor boost

Instructions:

1. **Blend the Base:**

   - In a blender, combine the frozen fruits, Greek yogurt, protein powder, and liquid. Blend until smooth and creamy. Adjust the liquid as needed to achieve your desired consistency.

2. **Pour into a Bowl:**
   - Fill a bowl with the smoothie mixture. The thickness should be similar to soft-serve ice cream.

3. **Add Toppings:**
   - Arrange your chosen toppings on the smoothie surface. Get creative with the arrangement to make your bowl visually appealing.

4. **Enjoy:**
   - Grab a spoon and enjoy your protein-packed smoothie bowl! Make sure to mix the toppings with the smoothie base for a variety of flavors and textures in each bite.

Tips:

- Experiment with different fruit combinations to find your favorite flavor profile.
- If desired, adjust the sweetness by drizzling in some honey or maple syrup.
- Consider adding a handful of spinach or kale to sneak in some leafy greens without affecting the taste.

This protein-packed smoothie bowl is not only a tasty treat but also a well-rounded breakfast that provides a mix of macronutrients to keep you energized throughout the morning.

HEARTY OMELETS AND EGG CREATION

Creating hearty omelets and egg-based creations allows for a versatile and satisfying breakfast or brunch. Here's a guide to making a hearty omelet and a few creative egg-based variations:

Classic Hearty Omelet:

Ingredients:

1. 2-3 large eggs
2. Salt and pepper to taste
3. 1 tablespoon butter or cooking oil
4. Filling options:
   - Diced bell peppers
   - Diced onions
   - Sliced mushrooms
   - Diced tomatoes
   - feta, cheddar, or any other type of grated cheese

Instructions:

1. **Prepare Ingredients:**
   - Dice and prepare your chosen vegetables and cheese.

2. **Whisk Eggs:**
   - Beat the eggs together in a bowl until fully blended. Season with salt and pepper.

3. **Cook Vegetables:**
   - In a non-stick skillet, heat butter or oil over medium heat. Add the diced vegetables and sauté until softened.

4. **Pour Eggs:**
   - Cover the sautéed veggies in the skillet with the whisked eggs.

5. **Swirl and Cook:**
   - Tilt the skillet to ensure the eggs spread evenly. As the edges set, gently lift them with a spatula, allowing the uncooked eggs to flow underneath.

6. **Add Cheese and Fold:**
   - Once the eggs are mostly set but still slightly runny on top, add your choice of cheese and fold the omelet in half.

7. **Serve:**
   - Slide the omelet onto a plate, and it's ready to be served. Garnish with fresh herbs if desired.

Creative Egg Creations: "Egg Muffins"

Ingredients:

1. 6 large eggs

2. Salt and pepper to taste
3. Filling options:
   - Diced ham or turkey
   - Chopped spinach
   - Diced bell peppers
   - Shredded cheese

Instructions:

1. **Preheat Oven:**
   - Set the oven temperature to 375°F, or 190°C.

2. **Whisk Eggs:**
   - In a bowl, whisk the eggs and season with salt and pepper.

3. **Prepare Muffin Tin:**
   - Use silicone muffin cups or grease a muffin tray.

4. **Add Fillings:**
   - Divide your chosen fillings among the muffin cups. Use your imagination to mix and match ingredients.

5. **Pour Eggs:**
   - Pour the whisked eggs over the fillings, filling each cup about 2/3 full.

6. **Bake:**
   - Bake in the preheated oven for 15-20 minutes or until the eggs are set.

7. **Serve:**
   - Before serving, let the egg muffins cool somewhat. You may eat them heated or room temperature.

These hearty omelets and egg muffins provide a protein-packed and customizable breakfast option. You are welcome to try a variety of fillings to suit your tastes.

ENERGIZING PROTEIN PANCAKES

Creating energizing protein pancakes is a delicious way to incorporate a protein boost into your breakfast. Here's a simple recipe for protein-packed pancakes:

Ingredients:

1. 1 cup of oats (quick oats or oat flour)
2. 1 ripe banana, mashed
3. 2 large eggs
4. 1/2 cup of Greek yogurt
5. 1 teaspoon baking powder
6. 1/2 teaspoon vanilla extract
7. Pinch of salt
8. Optional sweetener to taste (e.g., honey, maple syrup, or a sugar substitute)
9. Optional toppings: berries, sliced bananas, nuts, or a drizzle of nut butter

Instructions:

1. **Blend Oats:**
   - If using whole oats, blend them in a blender or food processor until you achieve a flour-like consistency.

2. **Mix Wet Ingredients:**
   - In a mixing bowl, combine the mashed banana, eggs, Greek yogurt, and vanilla extract. Mix well until smooth.

3. **Combine Dry Ingredients:**
   - Add the oat flour, baking powder, and a pinch of salt to the wet ingredients. Stir until just combined. Adjust the sweetness to your liking with optional sweeteners.

4. **Let Batter Rest:**
   - Allow the batter to rest for a few minutes. This helps the oats absorb some of the liquid, resulting in fluffier pancakes.

5. **Cook Pancakes:**
   - Increase the heat to medium in a griddle or nonstick skillet. Apply a tiny bit of butter or frying spray as a light grease.

   - Pour 1/4 cup portions of batter onto the skillet to form each pancake. Cook until surface bubbles appear, then turn and continue cooking until golden brown on the other side.

6. **Serve:**
   - Arrange the pancakes in a stack on a platter
and garnish with preferred ingredients. Fresh
berries, sliced bananas, nuts, or a drizzle of nut
butter are excellent choices.

7. **Enjoy:**
   - Serve the pancakes warm and enjoy your
energizing and protein-packed breakfast!

Tips:

- Experiment with adding a scoop of your favorite
protein powder to increase the protein content.
- Adjust the consistency of the batter by adding a
bit more liquid (milk or water) if needed.
- These pancakes can be customized with spices
like cinnamon or nutmeg for added flavor.

These energizing protein pancakes are not only
tasty but also provide a good balance of protein,
complex carbohydrates, and fiber to keep you
fueled throughout the morning.

CHAPTER FOUR

LUNCHTIME POWER PLATES

Crafting lunchtime power plates allows you to create well-balanced meals that provide sustained energy and essential nutrients. Here's a guide to building a nutritious and energizing lunch power plate:

GRILLED CHICKEN AND QUINOA SALAD

Certainly! Here's a simple recipe for Grilled Chicken and Quinoa Salad:

Ingredients:

For Grilled Chicken:

- 2 boneless, skinless chicken breasts
- Olive oil
- Lemon juice
- Salt and pepper
- Dried herbs, optional (try using oregano, thyme, or rosemary)

For Quinoa Salad:

- 1 cup quinoa, rinsed

- 2 cups water or chicken broth
- Cherry tomatoes, halved
- Cucumber, diced
- Red bell pepper, diced
- Red onion, finely chopped
- Fresh spinach or mixed greens
- Feta cheese, crumbled (optional)

For Dressing:

- 3 tablespoons olive oil
- 1 tablespoon balsamic vinegar
- 1 teaspoon Dijon mustard
- Salt and pepper to taste

Instructions:

Grilled Chicken:

1. Preheat the grill to medium-high heat.

2. In a bowl, mix olive oil, lemon juice, salt, pepper, and dried herbs (if using) to create a marinade.

3. Coat the chicken breasts with the marinade, ensuring they are well-covered.

4. Grill the chicken for 6-8 minutes per side or until fully cooked and has a nice char. A temperature of 165°F (74°C) should be reached internally.

5. Allow the chicken to rest for a few minutes before slicing it into strips.

Quinoa Salad:

1. In a saucepan, combine quinoa and water or chicken broth. Bring to a boil, then reduce heat, cover, and simmer for 15 minutes or until quinoa is cooked and liquid is absorbed.

2. Using a fork, fluff the quinoa and set aside to chill.

3. In a large bowl, combine the cooked quinoa, cherry tomatoes, cucumber, red bell pepper, red onion, and fresh spinach or mixed greens.

4. Add the grilled chicken strips to the salad.

Dressing:

1. In a small bowl, whisk together olive oil, balsamic vinegar, Dijon mustard, salt, and pepper.

2. Drizzle the dressing over the salad and toss gently until everything is well coated.

Assemble:

1. Sprinkle crumbled feta cheese over the top of the salad if desired.

2. Serve immediately, and enjoy your delicious
Grilled Chicken and Quinoa Salad!

Feel free to customize the salad with additional
ingredients like olives, avocado, or your favorite
herbs for added flavor and freshness.

LENTIL AND CHICKPEA BUDDHA BOWLS

Absolutely! Here's a simple recipe for Lentil and
Chickpea Buddha Bowls:

Ingredients:

For Lentils and Chickpeas:

- 1 cup dried lentils
- One can (15 oz) of rinsed and drained chickpeas
- Olive oil
- Garlic powder
- Cumin
- Smoked paprika
- Salt and pepper to taste

For Quinoa:

- 1 cup quinoa, rinsed
- 2 cups water or vegetable broth

For Vegetables:

- Sweet potatoes, peeled and cubed
- Broccoli florets
- Kale, destemmed and chopped
- Olive oil
- Salt and pepper

For Tahini Sauce:

- 1/4 cup tahini
- 2 tablespoons lemon juice
- 1 clove garlic, minced
- Salt and pepper to taste
- Water (to thin the sauce, if needed)

Instructions:

Lentils and Chickpeas:

1. Rinse the lentils and cook them according to package instructions. Set aside.

2. In a pan, heat olive oil over medium heat. Add chickpeas, garlic powder, cumin, smoked paprika, salt, and pepper. Sauté until the chickpeas are lightly browned. Set aside.

Quinoa:

1. In a saucepan, combine quinoa and water or vegetable broth. Bring to a boil, then reduce heat, cover, and simmer for 15 minutes or until quinoa is cooked. Using a fork, fluff and set aside.

Vegetables:

1. Preheat the oven to 400°F (200°C).

2. Toss sweet potatoes with olive oil, salt, and pepper. Simmer the potatoes for 20 to 25 minutes, or until they are soft.

3. Toss broccoli with olive oil, salt, and pepper. Add it to the baking sheet with sweet potatoes for the last 15 minutes of roasting.

4. In a pan, sauté chopped kale with olive oil until wilted. Season with salt and pepper.

Tahini Sauce:

1. In a small bowl, whisk together tahini, lemon juice, minced garlic, salt, and pepper. If the sauce is too thick, add water gradually until you achieve the desired consistency.

Assemble Buddha Bowls:

1. Divide cooked quinoa among bowls.

2. Arrange lentils, chickpeas, roasted sweet potatoes, broccoli, and sautéed kale on top of the quinoa.

3. Drizzle each bowl with tahini sauce.

4. Serve immediately and enjoy your nutritious Lentil and Chickpea Buddha Bowls!

Feel free to customize your Buddha bowls with additional toppings like avocado slices, cherry tomatoes, or a sprinkle of sesame seeds.

TURKEY AND AVOCADO WRAP

Certainly! Here's a simple and delicious recipe for a Turkey and Avocado Wrap:

Ingredients:

- 1 large whole wheat or spinach tortilla
- 4 oz sliced turkey breast
- 1/2 avocado, sliced
- 1/4 cup cherry tomatoes, halved
- 1/4 cup cucumber, thinly sliced
- Handful of fresh spinach leaves
- 1 tablespoon hummus (optional)
- Salt and pepper to taste

Instructions:

1. Lay the tortilla flat on a clean surface or plate.

2. If using hummus, spread it evenly over the tortilla, leaving a border around the edges.

3. Layer the sliced turkey evenly across the center of the tortilla.

4. Place avocado slices, cherry tomatoes, and cucumber on top of the turkey.

5. Add a handful of fresh spinach leaves on top of the vegetables.

6. Season with salt and pepper to taste.

7. If desired, you can drizzle a little extra virgin olive oil or your favorite dressing for added flavor.

8. Carefully fold the sides of the tortilla over the filling, and then roll it tightly from the bottom, creating a wrap.

9. Slice the wrap in half diagonally for easier handling.

10. Serve immediately, and enjoy your Turkey and Avocado Wrap!

Feel free to customize the wrap with additional ingredients like shredded cheese, red onion, or your favorite condiments. This quick and healthy wrap makes for a satisfying and balanced meal.

CHAPTER FIVE

DINNER DELIGHTS

Creating a delightful dinner involves balancing flavors, textures, and nutritional value. Here's a detailed explanation of dinner delights recipes:

SALMON WITH LEMON DILL SAUCE

Absolutely! Here's a simple and delicious recipe for Salmon with Lemon Dill Sauce:

Ingredients:

For Salmon:

- 4 salmon fillets
- Olive oil
- Salt and pepper to taste
- Lemon slices for garnish (optional)

For Lemon Dill Sauce:

- 1/2 cup plain Greek yogurt
- 1 tablespoon fresh dill, chopped
- 1 tablespoon lemon juice
- 1 teaspoon Dijon mustard

- 1 clove garlic, minced
- Salt and pepper to taste

Instructions:

For Salmon:

1. **Preheat Oven:** Preheat the oven to 375°F (190°C).

2. **Season Salmon:** Place the salmon fillets on a baking sheet lined with parchment paper. Add a drizzle of olive oil and season with pepper and salt. Ensure both sides are coated evenly.

3. **Bake Salmon:** Bake the salmon in the preheated oven for 15-20 minutes or until the salmon easily flakes with a fork. Depending on the thickness of the fillets, cooking times can change.

4. **Broil for Crispy Top (Optional):** If you desire a slightly crispy top, you can broil the salmon for an additional 2-3 minutes until the top is golden.

5. **Garnish (Optional):** Garnish with lemon slices for an extra burst of freshness.

For Lemon Dill Sauce:

1. **Prepare Sauce:** In a small bowl, whisk together Greek yogurt, chopped dill, lemon juice,

Dijon mustard, minced garlic, salt, and pepper.
Adjust the seasoning to taste.

2. **Serve:** Spoon the Lemon Dill Sauce over the
baked salmon fillets or serve it on the side.

3. **Garnish (Optional):** Garnish with additional
fresh dill for a visually appealing presentation.

4. **Enjoy:** Serve immediately, and enjoy your
Salmon with Lemon Dill Sauce!

Tips:

- This Lemon Dill Sauce not only complements
salmon but can also be used with other fish
varieties or grilled chicken.
- Feel free to customize the sauce by adjusting the
amount of lemon juice, dill, or garlic to suit your
taste preferences.

This recipe provides a perfect balance of the rich,
flaky salmon and the bright, herb-infused Lemon
Dill Sauce, creating a delightful and flavorful meal.

LEAN BEEF STIR-FRY

Certainly! Here's a simple and healthy recipe for
Lean Beef Stir-Fry:

Ingredients:

For Beef Marinade:

- 1 pound lean beef strips (sirloin or flank steak)
- 2 tablespoons soy sauce (low-sodium)
- 1 tablespoon oyster sauce
- 1 tablespoon rice vinegar
- 1 tablespoon cornstarch
- 1 teaspoon sesame oil
- 1 teaspoon grated ginger
- 2 cloves garlic, minced
- Freshly ground black pepper

For Stir-Fry:

- 1 tablespoon vegetable oil
- 1 onion, thinly sliced
- 1 bell pepper, thinly sliced (use a mix of colors for visual appeal)
- 1 cup broccoli florets
- 1 carrot, julienned
- 2 cups snap peas or snow peas, ends trimmed
- Cooked brown rice or quinoa for serving

Optional Garnish:

- Sesame seeds
- Green onions, sliced

Instructions:

Beef Marinade:

1. **Prepare Marinade:** In a bowl, combine soy sauce, oyster sauce, rice vinegar, cornstarch, sesame oil, grated ginger, minced garlic, and black pepper.

2. **Marinate Beef:** Place the lean beef strips in a Ziploc bag or shallow dish, and pour the marinade over the beef. Seal the bag or cover the dish and let it marinate in the refrigerator for at least 30 minutes to allow the flavors to infuse.

Stir-Fry:

1. **Heat Wok or Skillet:** In a wok or large skillet, heat vegetable oil over medium-high heat.

2. **Cook Beef:** Remove the beef from the marinade, allowing excess marinade to drip off. Stir-fry the beef in the hot wok for 2-3 minutes until browned and cooked through. After taking the steak out of the wok, set it aside.

3. **Cook Vegetables:** In the same wok, add a bit more oil if needed. Stir-fry the onion, bell pepper, broccoli, carrot, and snap peas for 3-4 minutes until the vegetables are crisp-tender but still vibrant.

4. **Combine and Toss:** Add the cooked beef back into the wok with the vegetables. Mix everything together until thoroughly hot and properly mixed.

5. **Serve:** Serve the lean beef stir-fry over cooked brown rice or quinoa.

Optional Garnish:

1. **Sprinkle Sesame Seeds:** Garnish with sesame seeds for added crunch and a nutty flavor.

2. **Top with Green Onions:** Finish with sliced green onions for a fresh and oniony kick.

Enjoy your delicious and nutritious Lean Beef Stir-Fry! This recipe provides a balance of protein, fiber, and vegetables for a satisfying and wholesome meal.

VEGETARIAN PROTEIN CASSEROLE

Certainly! Here's a tasty recipe for a Vegetarian Protein Casserole:

Ingredients:

For Casserole:

- 2 cups cooked quinoa or brown rice
- One can (15 oz) of rinsed and drained black beans
- One cup of fresh, frozen, or canned corn kernels
- 1 cup diced bell peppers (use a mix of colors)
- 1 cup cherry tomatoes, halved

- 1 cup shredded cheese (cheddar, Monterey Jack,
or a blend)
- 1 cup Greek yogurt or sour cream
- 1 teaspoon cumin
- 1 teaspoon chili powder
- Salt and pepper to taste

For Topping:

- 1 cup crushed tortilla chips or panko breadcrumbs
- 1/2 cup shredded cheese
- Fresh cilantro, chopped, for garnish

Instructions:

1. **Preheat Oven:** Preheat the oven to 375°F
(190°C).

2. **Prepare Casserole Mixture:**
   - In a large bowl, combine cooked quinoa or
brown rice, black beans, corn, diced bell peppers,
cherry tomatoes, shredded cheese, Greek yogurt or
sour cream, cumin, chili powder, salt, and pepper.
Blend thoroughly until all components are
dispersed equally.

3. **Transfer to Casserole Dish:**
   - Spread the mixture equally in a casserole dish
that has been buttered.

4. **Prepare Topping:**

   - In a separate bowl, mix crushed tortilla chips or panko breadcrumbs with shredded cheese.

5. **Top Casserole:**
   - Sprinkle the topping mixture evenly over the casserole.

6. **Bake:**
   - Bake in the preheated oven for 25-30 minutes or until the casserole is heated through, and the topping is golden brown and crispy.

7. **Garnish and Serve:**
   - Remove from the oven, garnish with fresh chopped cilantro, and let it cool slightly before serving.

8. **Serve Warm:**
   - Serve the Vegetarian Protein Casserole warm, and enjoy!

Tips:

- Customize the casserole by adding ingredients like diced avocado, green onions, or jalapeños for extra flavor.
- This casserole is versatile, and you can experiment with different types of beans, vegetables, or cheese according to your preferences.

This Vegetarian Protein Casserole offers a hearty and protein-packed dish that is not only delicious but also a great way to incorporate a variety of nutritious ingredients into your meal.

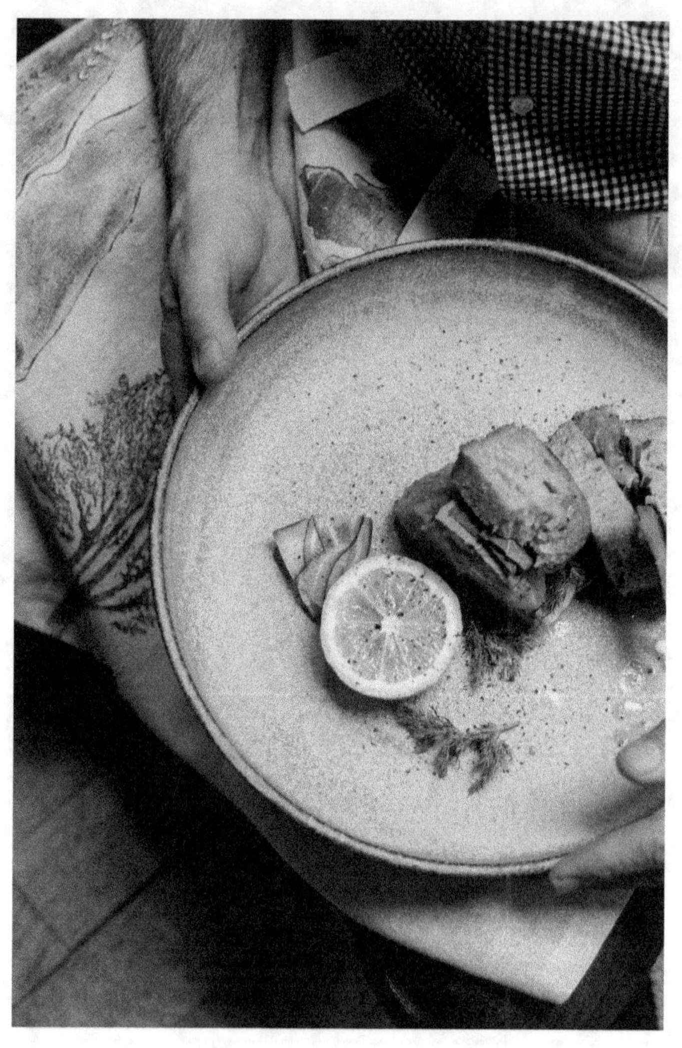

CHAPTER SIX

SNACK ATTACK: PROTEIN EDITION

Snack Attack: Protein Edition - Protein-Packed Greek Yogurt Parfait

Snacking doesn't have to be a guilty pleasure; it can be a delightful and nutritious experience, especially when it comes to incorporating protein into your snacks. Let's dive into a detailed explanation of creating a Protein-Packed Greek Yogurt Parfait, a satisfying and wholesome snack that balances flavor, texture, and nutritional value.

Ingredients:

Greek Yogurt Base:
- **1 cup Greek yogurt:** Opt for plain or your favorite flavored Greek yogurt. Greek yogurt is an excellent source of protein and provides a creamy base for the parfait.

Crunchy Layer:
- **1/4 cup granola:** Choose a granola variety that includes nuts and seeds for an extra protein boost and a satisfying crunch.

Berry Bliss:

- **1/2 cup mixed berries:** Incorporate a mix of berries like strawberries, blueberries, and raspberries. Berries not only add natural sweetness but also contribute vitamins and antioxidants.

Sweet Drizzle:
- **1 tablespoon honey or maple syrup:** Drizzle a touch of sweetness over the berries for added flavor. Adapt the quantity to your personal taste.

Nutrient-Rich Addition:
- **1 tablespoon chia seeds:** Sprinkle chia seeds over the honey or maple syrup. Chia seeds are rich in fiber and omega-3 fatty acids, offering additional nutritional benefits.

Optional Nut Topping:
- **Optional: a sprinkle of chopped nuts (almonds, walnuts):** For an extra protein boost and a delightful texture, add a sprinkle of your favorite chopped nuts.

Instructions:

1. **Layer Greek Yogurt:**
   - Begin by layering the bottom of a glass or bowl with Greek yogurt. The creamy texture of Greek yogurt provides a satisfying base for the parfait.

2. **Add Granola:**

- Scatter granola on top of the Greek yogurt. The granola adds a satisfying crunch and contributes to the protein content of the snack.

3. **Top with Mixed Berries:**
   - Add a generous layer of mixed berries on top of the granola. The combination of different berries introduces natural sweetness and various nutritional benefits.

4. **Drizzle with Honey or Maple Syrup:**
   - Drizzle honey or maple syrup over the berries to enhance the sweetness of the parfait. This step also adds a layer of indulgence to the snack.

5. **Sprinkle Chia Seeds:**
   - Sprinkle chia seeds over the honey or maple syrup. Chia seeds not only contribute to the overall texture but also bring in additional nutrients like fiber and omega-3 fatty acids.

6. **Optional Nut Topping:**
   - If you desire an extra protein boost and a delightful crunch, sprinkle a few chopped nuts over the top. This step is optional but adds a layer of richness to the parfait.

7. **Enjoy:**
   - Grab a spoon and savor each layer of your Protein-Packed Greek Yogurt Parfait. The combination of creamy yogurt, crunchy granola,

sweet berries, and nutritious seeds creates a
satisfying and delicious snack.

Tips:

- **Flavor Variations:** Experiment with different
flavors of Greek yogurt or add a splash of vanilla
extract for variety.

- **Fruit Choices:** Customize the parfait by
incorporating other fruits like sliced banana or kiwi
based on your preferences and seasonal
availability.

- **Granola Selection:** Choose a granola with
minimal added sugars for a healthier option. Look
for varieties that include nuts and seeds for added
nutritional value.

This Protein-Packed Greek Yogurt Parfait not only
addresses your snack cravings but also provides a
well-balanced mix of macronutrients, making it an
ideal choice for a tasty and nutritious snack. Enjoy
the layers of goodness in each bite!

NUT AND SEED TRAIL MIX

Certainly! Here's a simple recipe for a Nut and
Seed Trail Mix, a delightful and nutritious snack
that's perfect for on-the-go energy:

Ingredients:

- 1 cup almonds, raw or roasted
- 1 cup walnuts or pecans, raw or roasted
- 1/2 cup pumpkin seeds (pepitas)
- 1/2 cup sunflower seeds
- 1/2 cup cashews, raw or roasted
- 1/2 cup dried cranberries or raisins
- 1/4 cup chia seeds
- 1/4 cup flaxseeds (ground or whole)
- 1/4 cup dark chocolate chips or chunks (optional)
- 1 teaspoon cinnamon
- 1/2 teaspoon sea salt

Instructions:

1. **Prepare Nuts and Seeds:**
   - If using raw nuts, you can lightly toast them in a dry skillet over medium heat for a few minutes until they become fragrant. Allow them to cool before mixing.

2. **Mix Nuts and Seeds:**
   - In a large bowl, combine almonds, walnuts or pecans, pumpkin seeds, sunflower seeds, cashews, dried cranberries or raisins, chia seeds, flaxseeds, and dark chocolate chips (if using).

3. **Season with Cinnamon and Salt:**
   - Sprinkle cinnamon and sea salt over the mixture. Adjust the amount of cinnamon and salt based on your taste preferences.

4. **Toss to Combine:**
   - Gently mix all the ingredients until thoroughly mixed. Ensure an even distribution of nuts, seeds, and other add-ins.

5. **Store in an Airtight Container:**
   - Transfer the trail mix to an airtight container for storage. This makes it easy to grab a handful whenever you need a quick and nutritious snack.

6. **Enjoy On-The-Go:**
   - Grab a handful of your Nut and Seed Trail Mix whenever you're in need of a convenient and energy-boosting snack. It's great for hiking, commuting, or any time you're on the move.

Tips:

- **Customization:** Feel free to customize your trail mix by adding other nuts, seeds, or dried fruits based on your preferences.

- **Portion Control:** While trail mix is a nutritious snack, be mindful of portion sizes as nuts and seeds are calorie-dense. Pre-portioning into snack-sized bags can help with mindful snacking.

- **Allergy Considerations:** Adjust the ingredients to accommodate any nut or seed allergies, ensuring a safe and enjoyable snack for everyone.

This Nut and Seed Trail Mix is not only delicious but also packed with a variety of nutrients from nuts, seeds, and dried fruits, making it a wholesome and energizing snack option.

PROTEIN ENERGY BITES

Certainly! Here's a simple recipe for Protein Energy Bites, a nutritious and convenient snack that's easy to make:

Ingredients:

- 1 cup old-fashioned oats
- 1/2 cup nut butter (peanut butter, almond butter, or your choice)
- 1/3 cup honey or maple syrup
- 1/2 cup protein powder (vanilla or chocolate flavor works well)
- 1/2 cup ground flaxseeds
- 1 teaspoon vanilla extract
- A pinch of salt
- Optional add-ins: dark chocolate chips, chopped nuts, dried fruit

Instructions:

1. **Combine Dry Ingredients:**
   - In a large bowl, combine old-fashioned oats, protein powder, ground flaxseeds, and a pinch of salt. Stir until well mixed.

2. **Add Wet Ingredients:**
   - Add nut butter, honey or maple syrup, and vanilla extract to the dry ingredients. Mix thoroughly until you have a sticky and well-combined mixture.

3. **Optional Add-Ins:**
   - If desired, add in optional ingredients like dark chocolate chips, chopped nuts, or dried fruit. Taste and texture can be improved with these additions.

4. **Chill the Mixture:**
   - Refrigerate the mixture for approximately half an hour. Chilling makes it easier to shape the mixture into bites.

5. **Shape into Bites:**
   - After the mixture has cold, take small quantities and use your hands to roll them into bite-sized balls. The size is up to your preference, but typically, they are about one inch in diameter.

6. **Store:**
   - Place the protein energy bites on a plate or tray lined with parchment paper. Refrigerate them in an airtight container.

7. **Enjoy:**
   - Your Protein Energy Bites are ready to enjoy! They make for a quick and convenient snack, especially when you need an energy boost.

Tips:

- **Protein Powder:** Choose a protein powder that complements the flavor of your nut butter. Vanilla or chocolate protein powder works well in this recipe.

- **Texture Preference:** If you prefer a smoother texture, you can use instant oats instead of old-fashioned oats.

- **Customization:** Get creative with add-ins! Try dried cranberries, chopped almonds, or a sprinkle of shredded coconut for extra flavor.

These Protein Energy Bites are not only delicious but also packed with protein, fiber, and healthy fats, making them a great choice for a quick and nutritious snack.

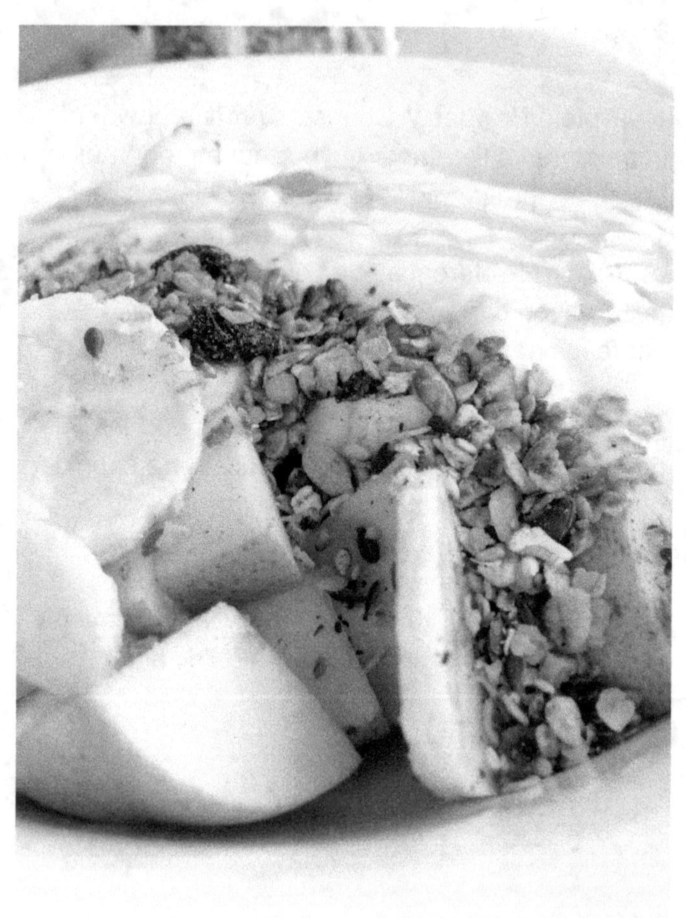

CHAPTER SEVEN

VEGETARIAN AND VEGAN VARIETIES

Vegetarian and Vegan Varieties: Nut and Seed Trail Mix

Vegetarian Nut and Seed Trail Mix:

Ingredients:
- Almonds, walnuts or pecans, pumpkin seeds, sunflower seeds, cashews, dried cranberries or raisins, chia seeds, flaxseeds, dark chocolate chips (optional), cinnamon, sea salt.

Instructions:
1. Combine all the ingredients following the provided quantities and instructions.
2. Ensure any optional add-ins, like chocolate chips, comply with vegetarian preferences.
3. Enjoy this vegetarian-friendly, protein-packed trail mix as a flavorful and energizing snack.

Vegan Nut and Seed Trail Mix:

Ingredients:
- Almonds, walnuts or pecans, pumpkin seeds, sunflower seeds, cashews, dried cranberries or

raisins, chia seeds, flaxseeds, dairy-free dark chocolate chips (optional), cinnamon, sea salt.

Instructions:
1. Follow the instructions for combining ingredients, replacing any non-vegan components with plant-based alternatives.
2. Ensure all ingredients, especially chocolate chips, are labeled as vegan or dairy-free.
3. Savor this vegan trail mix for a delicious and cruelty-free snack option.

Vegetarian and Vegan Varieties: Protein Energy Bites

Vegetarian Protein Energy Bites:

Ingredients:
- Old-fashioned oats, nut butter (peanut, almond, etc.), honey or maple syrup, vegetarian-friendly protein powder, ground flaxseeds, vanilla extract, pinch of salt, optional add-ins (dark chocolate chips, chopped nuts, dried fruit).

Instructions:
1. Combine the listed ingredients following the provided quantities and instructions.
2. Use a vegetarian-friendly protein powder for this variation.
3. Enjoy these vegetarian protein energy bites as a quick and nutritious snack.

Vegan Protein Energy Bites:

Ingredients:
- Old-fashioned oats, nut butter (peanut, almond, etc.), maple syrup or agave nectar, plant-based protein powder, ground flaxseeds, vanilla extract, pinch of salt, optional add-ins (dairy-free dark chocolate chips, chopped nuts, dried fruit).

Instructions:
1. Substitute honey with maple syrup or agave nectar for this vegan variation.
2. Ensure all ingredients, including protein powder and chocolate chips, are vegan-friendly.
3. Relish these vegan protein energy bites as a tasty and cruelty-free snack.

Tips for Both Varieties:
- Experiment with additional add-ins based on personal preferences.
- Consider portion control for mindful snacking, especially with energy-dense ingredients.
- Store in airtight containers for convenient access to these wholesome snacks.

These variations cater to different dietary preferences, offering flavorful and nutrient-packed options for both vegetarian and vegan individuals. Enjoy the goodness of nuts, seeds, and plant-based protein in these delightful trail mixes and energy bites!

TOFU AND VEGETABLE SKEWERS

Certainly! Here's a delicious recipe for Tofu and Vegetable Skewers:

Ingredients:

For Marinade:

- 1/4 cup soy sauce (low-sodium)
- 2 tablespoons olive oil
- 2 tbsp maple syrup (or agave nectar)
- 1 tablespoon rice vinegar
- 1 teaspoon minced garlic
- 1 teaspoon minced ginger
- 1 teaspoon sesame oil
- Salt and pepper to taste

For Skewers:

- 1 firm tofu block, squeezed and cut into cubes
- Cut one red bell pepper into pieces.
- One yellow bell pepper, chopped into pieces
- 1 zucchini, sliced into rounds
- 1 red onion, cut into wedges
- Cherry tomatoes
- Wooden skewers, soaked in water for at least 30 minutes

Instructions:

Marinating Tofu:

1. **Prepare Marinade:** In a bowl, whisk together soy sauce, olive oil, maple syrup or agave nectar, rice vinegar, minced garlic, minced ginger, sesame oil, salt, and pepper.

2. **Press Tofu:** Press the tofu to remove excess water. Cut the tofu into cubes.

3. **Marinate Tofu:** Place tofu cubes in a shallow dish and pour half of the marinade over them. Let it marinate for at least 30 minutes, turning the tofu occasionally for an even coating.

Assembling Skewers:

4. **Preheat Grill or Oven:** Preheat your grill or oven to medium-high heat.

5. **Assemble Skewers:** Thread marinated tofu cubes, bell pepper chunks, zucchini rounds, red onion wedges, and cherry tomatoes onto the soaked wooden skewers, alternating the ingredients.

Grilling Skewers:

6. **Grill Skewers:** Place the assembled skewers on the preheated grill. Grill for about 10-15 minutes, turning occasionally and basting with the remaining marinade until the tofu and vegetables are cooked and have a nice char.

Oven Option:

6. **Bake Skewers:** If using the oven, place skewers on a baking sheet lined with parchment paper. Bake at 400°F (200°C) for 20-25 minutes or until tofu and vegetables are cooked.

Serving:

7. **Serve Warm:** Once cooked, remove the skewers from the grill or oven. Serve the Tofu and Vegetable Skewers warm.

Tips:

- Customize the vegetables based on your preferences. Mushrooms, cherry tomatoes, and colorful bell peppers work well.
- For a full supper, serve the skewers with a side salad or rice.

These Tofu and Vegetable Skewers are not only a feast for the eyes but also a delicious and protein-packed dish that's perfect for a barbecue, outdoor gathering, or a flavorful weeknight dinner.

BLACK BEAN AND SWEET POTATO CHILI

Certainly! Here's a delicious recipe for Black Bean and Sweet Potato Chili:

Ingredients:

- 2 tablespoons olive oil
- 1 onion, chopped
- 3 cloves garlic, minced
- One big sweet potato, chopped and skinned
- 1 red bell pepper, chopped
- 1 yellow bell pepper, chopped
- Remove the seeds from one jalapeño and cut it finely (optional for heat).
- 2 teaspoons ground cumin
- 1 teaspoon chili powder
- 1/2 teaspoon smoked paprika
- 1/2 teaspoon ground cinnamon
- Salt and pepper to taste
- One can (15 oz) of rinsed and drained black beans
- One can (15 oz) of rinsed and drained black beans
- 2 cups vegetable broth
- One cup of fresh, frozen, or canned corn kernels
- Juice of 1 lime
- Fresh cilantro, chopped (for garnish)
- Avocado slices (for garnish)
- Greek yogurt or dairy-free yogurt (optional, for serving)

Instructions:

1. **Sauté Aromatics:**

- Heat the olive oil in a big pot over medium heat. Add chopped onion and garlic. Sauté until onions are translucent.

2. **Add Vegetables:**
   - Add diced sweet potato, red bell pepper, yellow bell pepper, and jalapeño (if using). Cook until the vegetables start to soften, about 5 to 7 minutes.

3. **Seasoning:**
   - Stir in ground cumin, chili powder, smoked paprika, ground cinnamon, salt, and pepper. Apply the spices to the vegetables in an equal layer.

4. **Combine Black Beans and Tomatoes:**
   - Add black beans, diced tomatoes (with their juice), and vegetable broth to the pot. Stir well to combine.

5. **Simmer:**
   - After bringing the chili to a simmer, turn down the heat. Cover and let it simmer for 20-25 minutes, allowing the flavors to meld and the sweet potatoes to become tender.

6. **Add Corn and Lime Juice:**
   - Add the lime juice and corn kernels and stir. Cook for an additional 5 minutes.

7. **Adjust Seasoning:**
   - Taste and correct the seasoning, adding extra spices, salt, or pepper as necessary.

8. **Serve:**
   - Ladle the chili into bowls. Garnish with fresh
cilantro, avocado slices, and a dollop of Greek
yogurt or dairy-free yogurt if desired.

Tips:

- Adjust the chili's thickness by adding more
vegetable broth if needed.
- For an extra protein boost, consider adding
cooked quinoa or serving the chili over rice.
- Customize the level of spiciness by adjusting the
amount of jalapeño or adding hot sauce to
individual servings.

This Black Bean and Sweet Potato Chili is a hearty
and flavorful dish that combines the sweetness of
sweet potatoes with the earthiness of black beans
and a blend of warm spices. Enjoy this comforting
chili on its own or with your favorite toppings.

QUINOA-STUFFED BELL PEPPERS

Certainly! Here's a tasty recipe for Quinoa-Stuffed
Bell Peppers:

Ingredients:

For Quinoa Stuffing:

- 1 cup quinoa, rinsed and cooked according to package instructions
- 1 tablespoon olive oil
- 1 onion, finely chopped
- 2 cloves garlic, minced
- 1 zucchini, diced
- 1 carrot, grated
- 1 cup cherry tomatoes, halved
- One can (15 oz) of rinsed and drained black beans
- 1 teaspoon ground cumin
- 1 teaspoon smoked paprika
- Salt and pepper to taste
- Juice of 1 lime
- Fresh cilantro, chopped (for garnish)

For Bell Peppers:

- Four huge bell peppers, seeded and halved
- Olive oil for brushing
- Salt and pepper to taste

Optional Toppings:

- Shredded cheese (cheddar or your choice)
- Avocado slices
- Sour cream or Greek yogurt

Instructions:

Preparing Quinoa Stuffing:

1. **Cook Quinoa:** Cook quinoa according to package instructions. Set aside.

2. **Sauté Vegetables:** In a large skillet, heat olive oil over medium heat. Add chopped onion and garlic. Sauté until onions are translucent.

3. **Add Zucchini and Carrot:** Add diced zucchini and grated carrot to the skillet. Cook the vegetables until they are soft, about 5 to 7 minutes.

4. **Combine Remaining Ingredients:** Stir in cooked quinoa, cherry tomatoes, black beans, ground cumin, smoked paprika, salt, and pepper. Cook for a further two to three minutes, or until well mixed.

5. **Finish with Lime Juice and Cilantro:** Squeeze lime juice over the quinoa mixture and stir in fresh cilantro. Remove from heat.

Preparing Bell Peppers:

6. **Preheat Oven:** Preheat the oven to 375°F (190°C).

7. **Prepare Bell Peppers:** Cut bell peppers in half lengthwise and remove seeds and membranes. Brush the outside of each pepper half with olive oil and season with salt and pepper.

8. **Stuff Peppers:** Fill each bell pepper half with the quinoa stuffing mixture, pressing down lightly.

9. **Bake:** Place stuffed bell peppers in a baking dish. Bake in the preheated oven for 25-30 minutes or until the peppers are tender.

10. **Optional Cheese Topping:** If desired, sprinkle shredded cheese over the stuffed peppers during the last 5 minutes of baking, allowing it to melt and slightly brown.

11. **Serve:** Remove from the oven and serve the quinoa-stuffed bell peppers hot.

Optional Toppings:

12. **Garnish:** Garnish with avocado slices, a dollop of sour cream or Greek yogurt, and additional fresh cilantro.

Tips:

- Feel free to experiment with different vegetables or add spices according to your taste preferences.
- Choose a mix of bell pepper colors for a visually appealing presentation.
- These stuffed peppers can be made ahead of time and reheated for convenience.

These Quinoa-Stuffed Bell Peppers are a nutritious and satisfying dish, combining the goodness of quinoa, black beans, and a variety of vegetables. Enjoy them as a wholesome meal or a flavorful side!

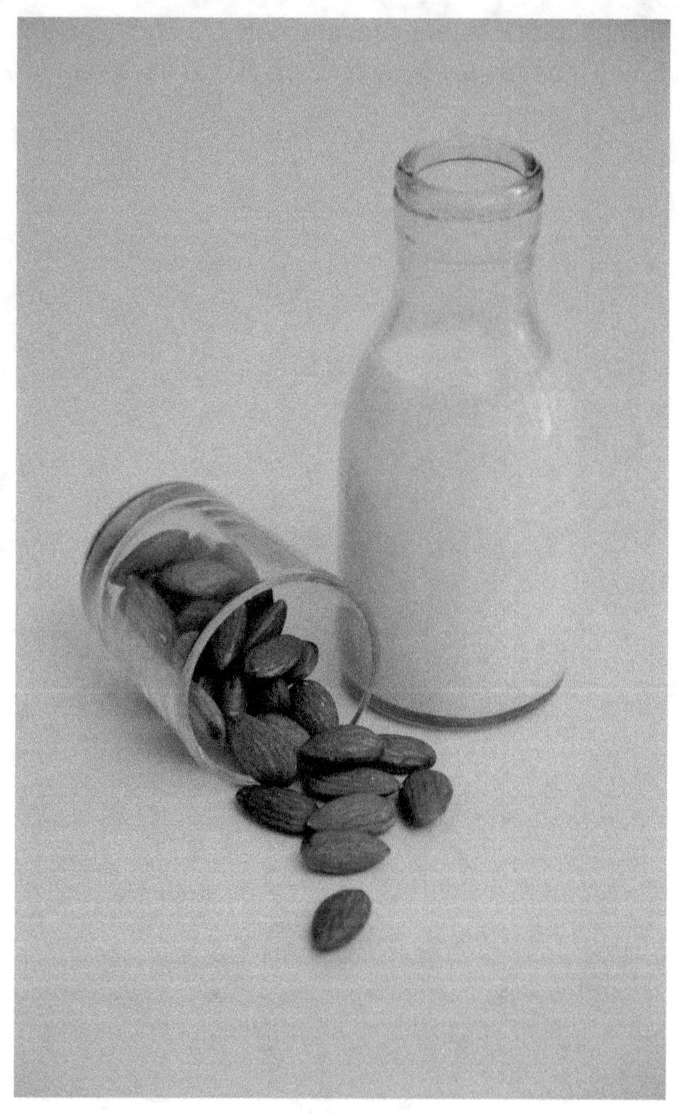

CHAPTER EIGHT

QUICK AND EASY PROTEIN FIXES

Certainly! Here are some quick and easy protein fixes that you can incorporate into your meals or snacks:

1. **Greek Yogurt Parfait:**
   - Layer Greek yogurt with granola, nuts, and berries for a protein-packed and delicious parfait.

2. **Hard-Boiled Eggs:**
   - Keep a batch of hard-boiled eggs in the fridge for a quick and portable protein snack.

3. **Protein Smoothie:**
   - Blend your favorite protein powder with almond milk, a banana, and a spoon of nut butter for a quick and tasty protein smoothie.

4. **Cottage Cheese and Fruit:**
   - Top a bowl of cottage cheese with fresh fruit or canned peaches for a simple and protein-rich snack.

5. **Nut Butter on Whole Grain Toast:**
   - Spread almond butter or peanut butter on whole grain toast for a quick and satisfying protein boost.

6. **Roasted Chickpeas:**
   - Toss chickpeas with olive oil and your favorite spices, then roast until crunchy for a tasty protein-packed snack.

7. **Turkey or Chicken Wraps:**
   - Wrap sliced turkey or chicken with your favorite veggies in a whole grain tortilla for a quick and portable protein fix.

8. **Cheese and Whole Grain Crackers:**
   - Pair cheese with whole grain crackers for a simple and satisfying protein-rich snack.

9. **Protein Bars:**
   - Keep a stash of protein bars in your bag for a convenient on-the-go protein fix.

10. **Tuna Salad Lettuce Wraps:**
    - Mix tuna with Greek yogurt, celery, and seasonings, then spoon it into lettuce leaves for a low-carb protein snack.

11. **Edamame:**
    - Enjoy steamed edamame sprinkled with sea salt for a tasty plant-based protein snack.

12. **Quinoa Salad:**
    - Toss cooked quinoa with veggies, beans, and a vinaigrette dressing for a quick and protein-packed salad.

13. **Hummus and Veggie Sticks:**
   - Dip sliced cucumbers, carrots, and bell peppers in hummus for a satisfying protein-rich snack.

14. **Beef Jerky:**
   - Keep a portion of lean beef jerky for a convenient and high-protein snack.

15. **Milk or Dairy Alternatives:**
   - Enjoy a glass of milk or a fortified dairy alternative for a quick and natural source of protein.

Remember to personalize these ideas based on your taste preferences and dietary requirements. These quick and easy protein fixes can be integrated into your daily routine for a balanced and nourishing diet.

20 MINUTE CHICKEN STIR-FRY

Certainly! Here's a quick and easy recipe for a 20-minute Chicken Stir-Fry:

Ingredients:

- One pound of finely sliced, boneless, skinless chicken breasts
- 2 tablespoons soy sauce (low-sodium)
- 1 tablespoon oyster sauce
- 1 tablespoon hoisin sauce

- 1 tablespoon sesame oil
- 1 tablespoon vegetable oil
- 3 cloves garlic, minced
- 1 tablespoon fresh ginger, grated
- 1 bell pepper, thinly sliced
- 1 cup broccoli florets
- 1 carrot, julienned
- 1 cup snap peas, ends trimmed
- 2 green onions, sliced (for garnish)
- Sesame seeds (for garnish, optional)
- Cooked rice or noodles (for serving)

Instructions:

1. **Prepare Ingredients:**
   - Slice chicken breasts thinly and prepare all vegetables before starting to ensure a quick cooking process.

2. **Marinate Chicken:**
   - In a bowl, combine sliced chicken with soy sauce, oyster sauce, and hoisin sauce. Allow it to marinate while you prepare the other ingredients.

3. **Heat Oils:**
   - In a wok or sizable skillet, heat the vegetable and sesame oils over medium-high heat.

4. **Sauté Chicken:**
   - Add the marinated chicken to the hot pan. Stir-fry for about 3-4 minutes until the chicken is

cooked through and slightly browned. Remove the chicken from the pan and set it aside.

5. **Sauté Aromatics:**
   - Add a little more oil to the same pan if necessary. Sauté minced garlic and grated ginger for about 30 seconds until fragrant.

6. **Cook Vegetables:**
   - Add bell pepper, broccoli, carrot, and snap peas to the pan. Vegetables should be stir-fried for 4–5 minutes to make them crisp-tender.

7. **Combine Chicken and Vegetables:**
   - Add the cooked chicken and veggies back to the pan. Toss everything together to combine.

8. **Adjust Seasoning:**
   - Taste and adjust the seasoning if needed. You can add a bit more soy sauce or a splash of water if it's too dry.

9. **Finish and Garnish:**
   - Remove from heat as soon as everything is well blended and heated through. If preferred, garnish with sesame seeds and sliced green onions.

10. **Serve:**
    - Serve noodles or cooked rice with the stir-fried chicken.

Tips:

- **Prep Ahead:** Cut and marinate the chicken in advance for an even quicker cooking process.
- **Vegetable Options:** Feel free to customize the vegetables based on what you have on hand or your preferences.
- **Spice it Up:** Add a pinch of red pepper flakes or sriracha if you like it spicy.

This quick and flavorful Chicken Stir-Fry is perfect for a speedy and delicious weeknight dinner. Adjust the ingredients to suit your taste, and enjoy the vibrant combination of tender chicken and crisp vegetables!

SPEEDY SHRIMP QUINOA BOWL

Certainly! Here's a quick and tasty recipe for a Speedy Shrimp Quinoa Bowl:

Ingredients:

For Quinoa:

- 1 cup quinoa, rinsed
- 2 cups water or vegetable broth
- Salt to taste

For Shrimp:

- One pound of big, peeled and deveined shrimp

- 1 tablespoon olive oil
- 2 cloves garlic, minced
- 1 teaspoon paprika
- Salt and pepper to taste
- Juice of 1 lemon

For Quinoa Bowl:

- 1 cup cherry tomatoes, halved
- 1 cucumber, diced
- 1 avocado, sliced
- 1/4 cup red onion, finely chopped
- Fresh cilantro, chopped (for garnish)
- Lime wedges (for serving)

Instructions:

Prepare Quinoa:

1. **Cook Quinoa:**
   - In a saucepan, combine quinoa, water or vegetable broth, and a pinch of salt. After bringing to a boil, lower the heat to a simmer, cover, and cook the quinoa for 15 to 20 minutes, or until it is tender and the water has been absorbed.

Prepare Shrimp:

2. **Season Shrimp:**
   - In a bowl, toss shrimp with minced garlic, paprika, salt, pepper, and lemon juice.

3. **Sauté Shrimp:**
   - Lightly heat the olive oil in a skillet over medium-high heat. Add the seasoned shrimp and cook for 2-3 minutes per side or until they are opaque and cooked through.

Assemble Quinoa Bowl:

4. **Fluff Quinoa:**
   - Using a fork, fluff the cooked quinoa.

5. **Serve Bowl:**
   - Divide quinoa among serving bowls.

6. **Top with Ingredients:**
   - Arrange cooked shrimp, cherry tomatoes, cucumber, avocado slices, and chopped red onion over the quinoa.

7. **Garnish:**
   - Garnish with fresh cilantro.

8. **Serve with Lime Wedges:**
   - Lime wedges should be served alongside for an added taste boost.

Tips:

- **Customize Vegetables:** Feel free to add or substitute vegetables based on your preferences. Bell peppers, corn, or spinach work well in this bowl.

- **Spice Level:** Adjust the level of paprika or add chili flakes if you prefer a spicier dish.
- **Protein Variation:** Swap shrimp for grilled chicken or tofu if you prefer.

This Speedy Shrimp Quinoa Bowl is not only quick to make but also a nutritious and flavorful meal. Enjoy the combination of protein-packed shrimp with fresh vegetables and fluffy quinoa!

NO-BAKE PROTEIN BARS

Certainly! Here's a simple recipe for No-Bake Protein Bars:

Ingredients:

- 1 cup old-fashioned oats
- One cup of protein powder, flavored to your liking
- 1/2 cup nut butter (peanut butter, almond butter, or your choice)
- 1/3 cup honey or maple syrup
- Half a cup of almond milk, or any other type of milk.
- 1 teaspoon vanilla extract
- A pinch of salt
- Optional add-ins: dark chocolate chips, chopped nuts, dried fruit

Instructions:

1. **Prepare Dry Ingredients:**

- Combine protein powder and oats in a big bowl.
Mix well.

2. **Warm Nut Butter and Sweetener:**
   - In a small saucepan over low heat, warm nut
butter and honey or maple syrup until they are easy
to stir.

3. **Combine Wet Ingredients:**
   - Stir in almond milk, vanilla extract, and a pinch
of salt into the warm nut butter and sweetener
mixture. Mix until well combined.

4. **Combine Wet and Dry Mixtures:**
   - Cover the dry ingredients with the wet mixture.
Till all of the dry ingredients are evenly covered,
thoroughly mix.

5. **Add Optional Ingredients:**
   - If desired, add dark chocolate chips, chopped
nuts, or dried fruit. Mix until evenly distributed.

6. **Press into Pan:**
   - Use parchment paper to line a square or
rectangular pan. Press the mixture firmly into the
pan, ensuring an even layer.

7. **Chill:**
   - Place the pan in the refrigerator for at least 2
hours, or until the mixture is firm.

8. **Cut into Bars:**

- Using the parchment paper, remove the bars
from the pan after they have cold. Place on a
cutting board and cut into bars of your desired size.

9. **Store:**
   - Store the bars in an airtight container in the
refrigerator for freshness. For simplicity, you can
also wrap each one separately.

Tips:

- **Customize Flavors:** Experiment with different
flavors of protein powder to create bars with your
favorite taste.
- **Texture Variation:** For a chewier texture, use
quick oats instead of old-fashioned oats.
- **Add Crunch:** For an extra crunch, include
crispy rice cereal in the mixture.
- **Make Them Nut-Free:** If you have nut
allergies, choose a nut-free butter (such as
sunflower seed butter) and skip nuts as add-ins.

These No-Bake Protein Bars are not only
convenient but also a nutritious snack option,
providing a good balance of protein, healthy fats,
and carbohydrates. Enjoy them as a quick
pick-me-up or a post-workout treat!

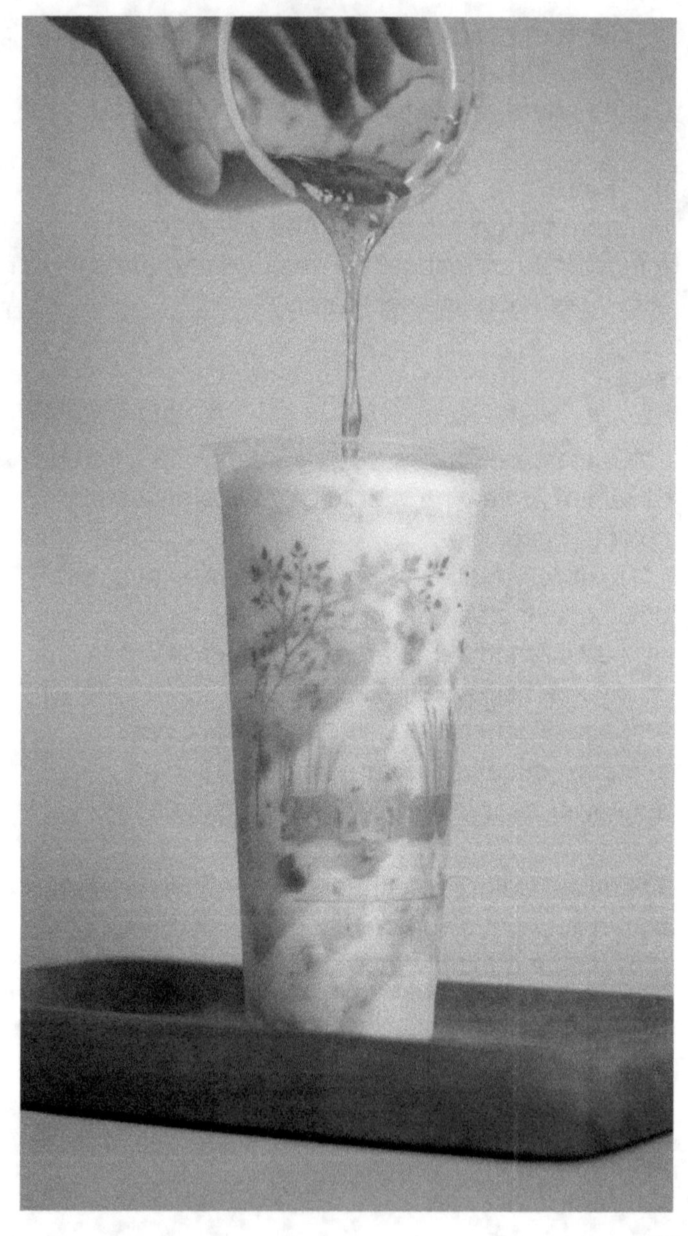

CHAPTER NINE

FITNESS FUEL

In the context of the "High Protein Cookbook for Women," the concept of fitness fuel takes on a nuanced and tailored significance. This section aims to provide women with a comprehensive understanding of how nutrition can be strategically employed to enhance their physical performance, promote recovery, and sustain overall well-being.

1. **Pre-Workout Preparation:**
   - *Objective:* Anticipating the energy demands of exercise and optimizing performance.
   - *Key Components:* Emphasis on complex carbohydrates for sustained energy release, moderate protein for muscle support, and incorporation of vitamins and minerals from whole foods.
   - *Examples:* Whole grain toast with almond butter and sliced banana or a yogurt parfait with granola and berries.

2. **Intra-Workout Hydration:**
   - *Objective:* Maintaining proper fluid balance and supporting electrolyte levels during exercise.
   - *Key Components:* Hydration through water or infused beverages, and consideration of electrolyte-rich options for longer or more intense workouts.

- *Examples:* Hydrating with water and a splash of lemon or enjoying a coconut water infused with electrolytes.

3. **Post-Workout Recovery:**
   - *Objective:* Facilitating muscle recovery, replenishing glycogen stores, and minimizing post-exercise fatigue.
   - *Key Components:* Prioritizing high-quality protein sources for muscle repair, carbohydrates to restore glycogen, and incorporating nutrient-dense vegetables for overall recovery.
   - *Examples:* Grilled chicken or tofu with quinoa and a variety of colorful roasted vegetables, or a protein smoothie with mixed berries and Greek yogurt.

4. **Protein Shakes and Smoothies Tailored for Women:**
   - *Objective:* Providing convenient and delicious options for protein intake, considering the unique nutritional needs of women.
   - *Key Components:* High-quality protein powder, nutrient-rich fruits or vegetables, and mindful consideration of macronutrient balance.
   - *Examples:* A protein smoothie with spinach, banana, and plant-based protein powder, or a shake with whey protein, mixed berries, and a touch of almond milk.

5. **High-Protein Recovery Snacks with a Feminine Touch:**

- *Objective:* Satisfying post-exercise hunger and supporting ongoing recovery between meals.
- *Key Components:* Protein-rich choices like Greek yogurt, nuts, or lean meats, paired with a source of carbohydrates and perhaps incorporating antioxidant-rich ingredients.
- *Examples:* Greek yogurt parfait with granola and mixed berries or a small serving of smoked salmon with whole-grain crackers.

Recognizing that women have unique nutritional needs due to hormonal fluctuations, reproductive health, and other factors, the "Fitness Fuel for Women" section in this cookbook seeks to empower women to engage in physical activity with confidence, knowing that their nutrition is specifically tailored to support their individual journeys. Each recipe is not just a meal but a deliberate step towards achieving holistic health, vitality, and strength.

PRE AND POST-WORKOUT NUTRITION

Pre and Post-Workout Nutrition for Women: Elevating Your Strength

In the "High Protein Cookbook for Women," pre and post-workout nutrition is a tailored and integral part of the culinary experience, designed to empower women on their fitness journey.

Pre-Workout Nutrition: Priming for Performance

1. **Timing is Everything:**
   - Plan your meal or snack 1-2 hours before exercising for optimal digestion.
   - For quick energy, consider a smaller snack 30 minutes prior to your workout.

2. **Carbohydrates for Steady Energy:**
   - Choose complex carbohydrates like quinoa, sweet potatoes, or whole-grain bread.
   - These provide sustained energy without causing rapid blood sugar spikes.

3. **Protein Boost for Muscle Support:**
   - Incorporate a moderate amount of high-quality protein to support muscle function and minimize muscle breakdown during exercise.
   - Options include Greek yogurt with berries, a small serving of grilled chicken, or a protein smoothie with added greens.

4. **Hydration with a Twist:**
   - Hydrate with water infused with a splash of citrus or a few slices of cucumber.
   - Consider coconut water for added electrolytes without added sugars.

Post-Workout Nutrition: Nourishing Your Recovery

1. **Swift Refueling within 30 Minutes:**
   - Consume a nutrient-rich meal or snack within 30 minutes of finishing your workout.
   - Optimize nutrient absorption during this crucial window.

2. **Protein Power for Recovery:**
   - Prioritize lean protein sources such as salmon, tofu, or beans to aid in muscle repair.
   - Enjoy a protein shake with almond milk and a handful of berries for a quick and convenient option.

3. **Carbohydrates for Glycogen Restoration:**
   - Include whole-food carbohydrates to replenish glycogen stores and support recovery.
   - Options may include quinoa salads, whole-grain wraps with lean protein, or a colorful fruit salad.

4. **Hydration and Rehydration:**
   - Continue to hydrate post-exercise to replace fluids lost during your workout.
   - Choose hydrating foods like water-rich fruits and vegetables.

5. **Antioxidant-Rich Additions:**
   - Integrate antioxidant-rich foods to combat oxidative stress.
   - Berries, dark chocolate, and nuts can enhance recovery while satisfying sweet cravings.

This personalized approach to pre and post-workout nutrition in the cookbook acknowledges the unique needs of women, considering factors such as hormonal fluctuations and reproductive health. Each recipe serves as a delicious and purposeful step towards empowering women to not only meet but surpass their fitness goals while savoring the journey to strength, vitality, and well-being.

PROTEIN SHAKES AND SMOOTHIES FOR ACTIVE WOMEN

Protein Shakes and Smoothies: Energizing Elixirs for Active Women

In the "High Protein Cookbook for Women," the chapter on protein shakes and smoothies is a celebration of delicious and nutritious blends designed to fuel the active lifestyles of women.

1. Berry Bliss Protein Smoothie:
  - *Ingredients:* Mixed berries, Greek yogurt, a scoop of protein powder, almond milk, and a handful of spinach.
  - *Benefits:* Packed with antioxidants, vitamins, and high-quality protein for muscle support.

2. Tropical Paradise Protein Shake:
  - *Ingredients:* Pineapple, mango, coconut water, protein powder, and a touch of chia seeds.

  - *Benefits:* Refreshing tropical flavors, hydrating coconut water, and a protein punch for post-workout recovery.

3. Green Goddess Power Smoothie:
  - *Ingredients:* Kale, banana, avocado, protein powder, and almond milk.
  - *Benefits:* Rich in greens, healthy fats, and protein for sustained energy and muscle repair.

4. Chocolate Peanut Butter Protein Shake:
  - *Ingredients:* Chocolate protein powder, peanut butter, banana, and milk of choice.
  - *Benefits:* A satisfying blend of chocolate and nutty goodness, delivering essential protein and healthy fats.

5. Energizing Espresso Protein Smoothie:
  - *Ingredients:* Cold brew coffee, protein powder, almond milk, a banana, and a dash of cinnamon.
  - *Benefits:* A caffeinated pick-me-up combined with protein for a pre or post-workout energy boost.

6. Creamy Coconut Almond Joy Shake:
  - *Ingredients:* Coconut milk, almond butter, protein powder, a hint of vanilla, and shredded coconut.
  - *Benefits:* Indulgent flavors reminiscent of a beloved candy bar, with the nutritional benefits of protein and healthy fats.

7. Mixed Nut Power Smoothie:

   - *Ingredients:* Mixed nuts (walnuts, almonds), banana, protein powder, and milk of choice.
   - *Benefits:* A nutty delight providing a mix of textures, flavors, and essential nutrients.

These protein shakes and smoothies are carefully crafted to cater to the specific nutritional needs of active women. Whether you're gearing up for a workout, replenishing after an exercise session, or simply seeking a nutritious and delicious snack, these recipes offer a delightful fusion of flavors while ensuring your body receives the protein it needs to thrive. Cheers to blending health, flavor, and vitality in every sip!

HIGH PROTEIN RECOVERY SNACKS

High-Protein Recovery Snacks: Nourishing Your Body, Renewing Your Energy

In the "High Protein Cookbook for Women," the chapter on high-protein recovery snacks is a treasure trove of delectable and nutrient-packed treats designed to support muscle recovery and keep you energized between meals.

1. Greek Yogurt Parfait:
   - *Ingredients:* Greek yogurt, honey, mixed berries, and a sprinkle of granola.
   - *Benefits:* Rich in protein, probiotics, and antioxidants for muscle recovery and digestive health.

2. Nutty Banana Protein Bites:
   - *Ingredients:* Mashed banana, almond butter, protein powder, and chopped nuts.
   - *Benefits:* A portable and satisfying snack providing a blend of protein, healthy fats, and natural sweetness.

3. Smoked Salmon and Avocado Rice Cakes:
   - *Ingredients:* Whole grain rice cakes, smoked salmon, mashed avocado, and a sprinkle of chia seeds.
   - *Benefits:* Omega-3 fatty acids, high-quality protein, and complex carbohydrates for a balanced and savory snack.

4. Quinoa Energy Balls:
   - *Ingredients:* Cooked quinoa, almond butter, honey, and dark chocolate chips.
   - *Benefits:* A bite-sized powerhouse combining protein, fiber, and energy-boosting ingredients.

5. Edamame and Roasted Chickpea Mix:
   - *Ingredients:* Edamame, roasted chickpeas, a drizzle of olive oil, and your favorite spices.
   - *Benefits:* A crunchy and savory blend rich in plant-based protein, fiber, and essential nutrients.

6. Cottage Cheese and Pineapple Cups:
   - *Ingredients:* Cottage cheese, fresh pineapple chunks, and a sprinkle of shredded coconut.

   - *Benefits:* High protein content, digestive enzymes from pineapple, and a touch of tropical sweetness.

7. Turkey and Hummus Stuffed Cucumber Boats:
   - *Ingredients:* Sliced cucumber, lean turkey slices, and a dollop of hummus.
   - *Benefits:* A low-carb, high-protein snack with the added benefits of hydration from cucumber.

These high-protein recovery snacks are not only delicious but also purposefully crafted to aid in muscle repair, replenish energy, and keep you fueled throughout the day. Whether enjoyed post-workout or as a satisfying midday pick-me-up, these snacks contribute to the holistic approach to health and well-being advocated in the cookbook. Indulge in these nutrient-packed delights, and let each bite be a step towards your journey to strength, vitality, and sustained energy.

CHAPTER TEN

MASTERING MEAL PREP

Mastering meal prep is a fantastic skill for saving time, maintaining a healthy diet, and reducing stress during the week. Here's a guide to help you become a meal prep pro:

1. **Plan Your Meals:**

- **Choose Recipes:** Select recipes that are easy to prepare, balanced, and can be stored well.

- **Consider Nutritional Needs:** Ensure your meals include a mix of protein, carbohydrates, healthy fats, and vegetables.

- **Create a Menu:** Take into account breakfast, lunch, dinner, and snacks while planning your weekly menu.

2. **Make a Grocery List:**

- **Check Pantry and Fridge:** Take stock of what you already have to avoid unecessary purchases.

- **Stick to the List:** Plan your shopping list based on your menu to avoid impulse buying.

3. **Batch Cooking:**

- **Choose Batch-Friendly Recipes:** Opt for recipes that can be easily multiplied, like casseroles, stews, or roasted vegetables.

- **Cook in Bulk:** Prepare larger quantities to have leftovers for multiple meals.

4. **Invest in Storage Containers:**

- **Choose the Right Containers:** Invest in a variety of containers suitable for storing different types of food.

- **Portion Control:** Use containers to pre-portion meals, making it easy to grab and go.

5. **Organize Your Kitchen:**

- **Clear Workspace:** Ensure you have ample space to work efficiently.

- **Organize Ingredients:** Arrange ingredients in a way that makes the cooking process seamless.

6. **Schedule Meal Prep Time:**

- **Set a Routine:** Choose a specific day and time each week for meal prep.

- **Start Small:** If you're new to meal prep, begin with a few recipes and gradually expand.

7. **Multitasking Tips:**

- **Utilize Oven and Stovetop:** Cook multiple items simultaneously to save time.

- **Prep Ingredients in Batches:** Chop vegetables, marinate proteins, or prepare grains in one go.

8. **Include Variety:**

- **Rotate Ingredients:** Keep your meals interesting by rotating proteins, grains, and vegetables.

- **Try New Recipes:** Experiment with new recipes to avoid mealtime monotony.

9. **Label and Date:**

- **Label Containers:** Clearly label containers with the contents and date of preparation.

- **Follow FIFO:** Practice "first in, first out" to use older meals before newer ones.

10. **Freezing Meals:**

- **Freezer-Friendly Recipes:** Identify recipes that freeze well for longer storage.

- **Portion for Freezing:** Portion meals before freezing for easier thawing and reheating.

11. **Reheating Tips:**

- **Use Microwave or Oven:** Reheat meals using microwave or oven for better texture.

- **Add Fresh Elements:** Add fresh herbs, greens, or a squeeze of citrus after reheating for added freshness.

12. **Stay Consistent:**

- **Make It a Habit:** Consistency is key. The more you meal prep, the easier it becomes.

- **Adapt as Needed:** Adjust your meal prep routine based on feedback and changing schedules.

13. **Enjoy the Benefits:**

- **Time-Saving:** Save time during the week by having meals ready to go.

- **Healthier Choices:** Ensure healthier choices by controlling ingredients and portions.

- **Financial Savings:** Save money by buying ingredients in bulk and reducing dining out.

Mastering meal prep takes practice, so don't be afraid to adapt and refine your process based on what works best for you. It will eventually become a smooth part of your daily routine.

WEEKLY MEAL PREP CALENDAR

Creating a meal prep calendar can help you stay organized and ensure a variety of meals throughout the week. Here's a sample meal prep calendar to get you started:

Week 1:

Monday:
- Breakfast: Berries and nuts in overnight oats
- Lunch: Chickpeas, cucumber, and feta in a quinoa salad
- Dinner: Baked lemon herb chicken with roasted sweet potatoes and broccoli

Tuesday:
- Breakfast: Greek yogurt parfait with granola and mixed fruits
- Lunch: Lentil and vegetable soup
- Dinner: Shrimp stir-fry with brown rice and mixed vegetables

Wednesday:
- Breakfast: Poached eggs and avocado on whole grain bread
- Lunch: Turkey and avocado wrap with a side of cherry tomatoes
- Dinner: Vegetarian chili with quinoa

Thursday:
- Breakfast: Protein smoothie with spinach, banana, and protein powder
- Lunch: With whole grain crackers, a caprese salad
- Dinner: quinoa-topped baked salmon served with steaming asparagus

Friday:
- Breakfast: Cottage cheese with pineapple and a sprinkle of chia seeds
- Lunch: Whole grain croutons paired with chicken Caesar salad
- Dinner: Stir-fried vegetables and beef over brown rice

Saturday:
- Breakfast: Scrambled eggs with spinach and whole grain toast
- Lunch: Hummus and veggie wraps
- Dinner: Marinara sauced spaghetti squash topped with turkey meatballs

Sunday:

- Breakfast: Protein pancakes with berries and a drizzle of maple syrup
- Lunch: Quinoa-stuffed bell peppers
- Dinner: Grilled chicken with quinoa and a side of roasted Brussels sprouts

Week 2:

Follow a similar pattern but switch up the protein sources, grains, and vegetables to keep things interesting.

Tips:

- **Rotate Ingredients:** Use different proteins (chicken, shrimp, beef, beans), grains (quinoa, brown rice, whole wheat pasta), and vegetables to create variety.

- **Prep in Batches:** On a designated day, batch-cook staples like quinoa, roasted vegetables, and proteins.

- **Portion Control:** Use portion-controlled containers to make grabbing meals easy.

- **Mix and Match:** Feel free to mix and match meals based on your preferences for each day.

- **Snack Prep:** Include healthy snacks like cut-up veggies with hummus, fruit, or Greek yogurt with nuts.

- **Stay Flexible:** Be open to adjusting the plan based on your schedule and preferences.

Remember to customize the calendar based on your dietary preferences, nutritional needs, and portion sizes. This template is a starting point, and you can adjust it to fit your tastes and lifestyle.

CHAPTER ELEVEN

NUTRITIONAL INSIGHTS

Certainly! Here are some nutritional insights to consider for a well-balanced and healthy lifestyle:

1. **Balance Macronutrients:**

- **Proteins:** Include lean sources like poultry, fish, beans, and tofu for muscle repair and overall body function.

- **Carbohydrates:** Opt for complex carbohydrates like whole grains, fruits, and vegetables for sustained energy.

- **Fats:** Choose healthy fats from sources like avocados, nuts, seeds, and olive oil for heart health.

2. **Portion Control:**

- **Mindful Eating:** Recognize portion sizes to prevent overindulging and encourage healthy weight management.

- **Use Smaller Plates:** Using smaller plates can help control portion sizes and prevent excessive calorie intake.

3. **Hydration:**

- **Water Intake:** Stay adequately hydrated by sipping plenty of water throughout the day. Aim for at least 8 glasses.

- **Limit Sugary Drinks:** Minimize the intake of sugary beverages like sodas and opt for water, herbal teas, or infused water.

4. **Diverse Nutrient Sources:**

- **Eat the Rainbow:** Consume a variety of colorful fruits and vegetables to ensure a diverse range of nutrients.

- **Include Whole Foods:** Focus on whole, minimally processed foods to maximize nutrient intake.

5. **Meal Timing:**

- **Regular Meals:** Aim for regular meals to maintain energy levels and prevent overeating later in the day.

- **Balanced Snacks:** Include balanced snacks with a mix of protein, fiber, and healthy fats to curb hunger.

6. **Mindful Eating:**

- **Enjoy Your Meals:** Eat slowly, savoring each bite. This helps you recognize fullness and promotes digestion.

- **Limit Distractions:** Avoid distractions like TV or screens during meals to stay connected with your eating experience.

7. **Nutrient-Dense Snacking:**

- **Healthy Snacks:** Choose nutrient-dense snacks such as Greek yogurt, nuts, seeds, or fresh fruit.

- **Plan Snacks:** Plan your snacks to avoid reaching for less nutritious options when hunger strikes.

8. **Limit Processed Foods:**

- **Read Labels:** Check food labels and limit intake of processed foods high in added sugars, salt, and unhealthy fats.

- **Cook at Home:** Cooking at home allows you to control ingredients and make healthier choices.

9. **Individualized Nutrition:**

- **Consider Dietary Preferences:** Tailor your diet to your individual preferences, whether vegetarian, vegan, or omnivorous.

- **Consider Health Conditions:** Adjust your diet based on any specific health conditions or dietary needs.

10. **Regular Physical Activity:**

- **Combine with Nutrition:** Regular exercise complements a healthy diet for overall well-being.

- **Find Enjoyable Activities:** Choose physical activities you enjoy to make exercise a sustainable part of your routine.

11. **Sleep and Stress Management:**

- **Adequate Sleep:** Prioritize good sleep hygiene for overall health and weight management.

- **Stress Reduction:** Practice stress-reducing activities like meditation, yoga, or deep breathing.

12. **Consult with Professionals:**

- **Nutritional Guidance:** Consider consulting with a registered dietitian or nutritionist for personalized advice.

- **Medical Advice:** For specific health concerns, consult with a healthcare professional for personalized guidance.

Remember, these insights are general recommendations, and individual needs may vary. It's always beneficial to consult with healthcare or nutrition professionals for personalized advice tailored to your unique circumstances.

UNDERSTANDING LABELS AND PORTION CONTROL

Understanding Labels:

1. **Serving Size:**
   - Pay attention to the serving size. It affects the number of calories and nutrients you are consuming.

2. **Calories:**
   - Check the total calories per serving. This helps you manage your overall daily calorie intake.

3. **Nutrient Content:**
   - Look for nutrients like protein, fiber, vitamins, and minerals. Aim for products rich in essential nutrients.

4. **% Daily Value (%DV):**
   - The %DV indicates how much a nutrient in a serving contributes to a daily diet. Aim for foods with higher %DV of essential nutrients.

5. **Limit Certain Nutrients:**

- Be mindful of nutrients to limit, such as saturated fat, trans fat, sodium, and added sugars. Choose products with lower amounts of these.

6. **Ingredient List:**
   - Materials are arranged by weight in descending order. aware of added sugars, unhealthy fats, and artificial additives.

7. **Allergen Information:**
   - Check for allergen information if you have food sensitivities or allergies.

8. **Claims and Marketing Terms:**
   - Be cautious with terms like "low-fat," "sugar-free," or "natural." They may not always indicate a healthier choice.

Portion Control:

1. **Use Measuring Tools:**
   - To measure servings precisely, use a food scale, measuring cups, or spoons.

2. **Visual Cues:**
   - Acquire the ability to gauge portion sizes based on visual clues. A dish of meat, for instance, is roughly the size of a deck of cards.

3. **Plate Composition:**
   - Divide your plate: half with vegetables, a quarter with protein, and a quarter with carbohydrates.

4. **Single Servings:**
   - Choose single-serving packages or pre-portion snacks to avoid overeating.

5. **Avoid Eating from the Container:**
   - Portion out servings onto a plate to avoid mindlessly eating directly from the package.

6. **Listen to Hunger Cues:**
   - Pay attention to hunger and fullness cues. Eat until you're content, not until you're too stuffed.

7. **Practice Mindful Eating:**
   - Eat without distractions, savor each bite, and be aware of the flavors and textures.

8. **Cook at Home:**
   - Cooking at home allows you to control portion sizes and ingredient choices.

9. **Beware of Restaurant Portions:**
   - Restaurant portions are often larger. Take into account bringing leftovers home or sharing dishes.

10. **Use Smaller Plates:**
    - Smaller plates can create the illusion of a larger portion, helping with portion control.

11. **Stay Hydrated:**
    - Drink water before meals to help control appetite and prevent overeating.

12. **Plan Ahead:**
   - Plan your meals and snacks in advance to avoid impulsive, oversized servings.

Remember, practicing portion control and understanding food labels are crucial components of maintaining a healthy and balanced diet. It's about making mindful choices to support your overall well-being.

BALANCING MACROS FOR OPTIMAL HEALTH

Balancing macros, which include proteins, carbohydrates, and fats, is essential for optimal health. Here's a guide on how to achieve a balanced macro intake:

1. **Proteins:**

- **Role in Health:**
  - Proteins are crucial for building and repairing tissues, supporting immune function, and creating enzymes and hormones.

- **Sources:**
  - Include lean meats, poultry, fish, eggs, dairy, legumes, tofu, and plant-based protein sources.

- **Ideal Intake:**

- Aim for 15-25% of your daily caloric intake to come from protein sources.

2. **Carbohydrates:**

- **Role in Health:**
  - Carbs are the body's primary energy source, supporting brain function, and providing fuel for physical activity.

- **Sources:**
  - Choose whole grains, fruits, vegetables, legumes, and starchy vegetables for complex carbohydrates.

- **Ideal Intake:**
  - Around 45-65% of your total daily calories should come from carbohydrates.

3. **Fats:**

- **Role in Health:**
  - Fats are essential for absorbing fat-soluble vitamins, supporting brain function, and providing a concentrated source of energy.

- **Sources:**
  - Choose healthy fats from avocados, nuts, seeds, olive oil, and fatty seafood.

- **Ideal Intake:**

- Approximately 20-35% of your daily calories should come from healthy fats.

Tips for Balancing Macros:

1. **Individual Needs:**
   - Adjust your macro ratios based on individual factors such as age, gender, activity level, and health goals.

2. **Whole Foods:**
   - Prioritize whole, minimally processed foods to ensure a broad spectrum of nutrients.

3. **Portion Control:**
   - Be mindful of portion sizes to avoid overeating and to maintain a balanced intake of macros.

4. **Meal Timing:**
   - Distribute your macro intake across meals to support sustained energy throughout the day.

5. **Nutrient Timing:**
   - Consider the timing of macros around workouts, emphasizing protein and carbohydrates for recovery.

6. **Hydration:**
   - Stay hydrated, as water plays a role in various metabolic processes and supports overall health.

7. **Listen to Your Body:**

- Pay attention to hunger and fullness cues. Eat till you're full and stop when you're done.

8. **Experiment and Adjust:**
   - Experiment with different macro ratios and adjust based on how your body responds and your health goals.

9. **Consider Dietary Preferences:**
   - Tailor your macronutrient intake to your dietary preferences, whether it's vegetarian, vegan, or omnivorous.

10. **Consult Professionals:**
   - Seek guidance from a registered dietitian or nutritionist for personalized advice based on your health needs.

Remember, achieving a balance of macros is about finding what works best for your body, lifestyle, and health goals. It's not a one-size-fits-all approach, and individual needs may vary.

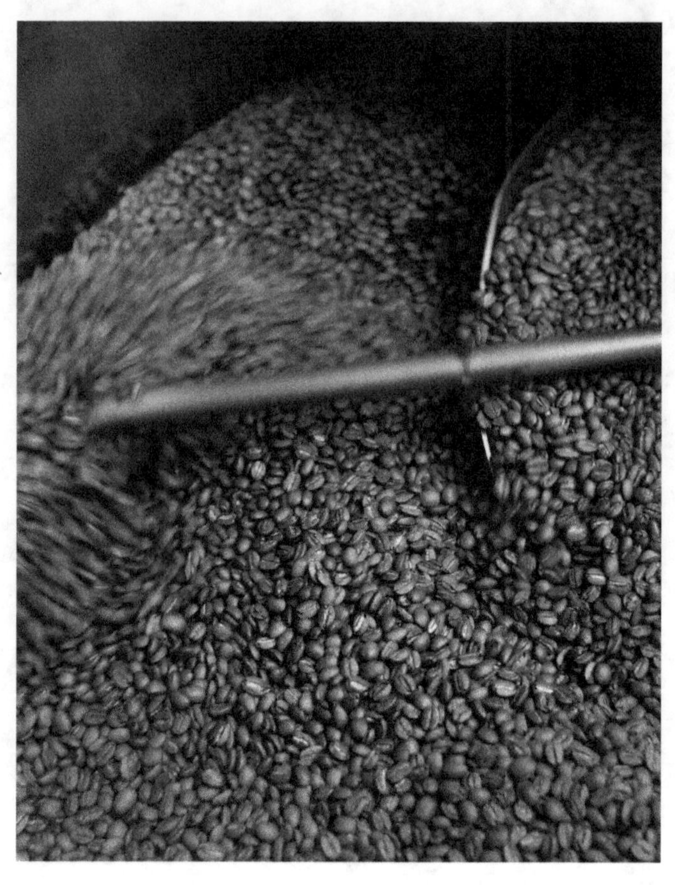

CHAPTER TWELVE

MINDFUL EATING AND PORTION CONTROL

Mindful Eating and Portion Control: Nourishing Your Body with Awareness

In the "High Protein Cookbook for Women," the marriage of mindful eating and portion control is a powerful combination, transforming your relationship with food into a conscious and balanced practice. Explore these principles to savor your meals with awareness while maintaining portion control for optimal well-being.

1. Begin with Mindful Awareness:
   - Before taking a bite, pause to cultivate awareness. Observe your feelings of hunger or fullness, and acknowledge the sensory aspects of your meal, from its aroma to its visual appeal.

2. Use Smaller Plates and Bowls:
   - Opt for smaller plates and bowls to naturally control portion sizes. This visual cue helps prevent overeating by providing a sense of satiety with a well-portioned plate.

3. Listen to Your Body:

- Be mindful of your body's signals of hunger and fullness. Eat solely when you're hungry and stop when you're full. Allow your body's natural cues to guide your portion sizes rather than relying on external cues.

4. Chew Slowly and Enjoy Every Bite:
   - Eat more slowly and enjoy every taste. Chewing slowly not only enhances the pleasure of eating but also allows your body to register fullness more effectively.

5. Mindful Beverage Consumption:
   - Be mindful of liquid calories and their impact on overall intake. Opt for water or other low-calorie beverages and savor them alongside your meal rather than mindlessly consuming high-calorie drinks.

6. Practice the 80/20 Rule:
   - Embrace the 80/20 rule, where you aim to eat until you're 80% full. This mindful approach leaves room for satisfaction without reaching the point of discomfort.

7. Eliminate Distractions:
   - Remove all distractions from the dining area to foster mindfulness. Put electronics away, turn off screens, and concentrate only on the process of eating. This enables you to fully appreciate the tastes and textures of your food.

8. Portion-Controlled Snacking:
   - Apply portion control to snacks by pre-portioning them into small containers. This helps prevent mindless munching and ensures that you're aware of the quantity you're consuming.

9. Use Visual Cues:
   - Use visual cues to estimate portion sizes. Familiarize yourself with recommended serving sizes for different food groups, allowing you to make more informed choices.

10. Practice Gratitude:
   - Cultivate gratitude for the nourishment your meal provides. Acknowledge the effort that went into preparing your food and express gratitude for the abundance on your plate.

By merging mindful eating with portion control, you foster a deeper connection with your body's signals and cultivate a balanced and enjoyable relationship with food. This harmonious approach not only supports your nutritional goals but also contributes to a positive and sustainable lifestyle.

BALANCING PROTEIN INTAKE WITH OTHER NUTRIENTS

Balancing Protein Intake with Other Nutrients: A Symphony of Nutrition

In the "High Protein Cookbook for Women," achieving a well-rounded and balanced diet involves more than just emphasizing protein. Explore these strategies to harmonize your protein intake with other essential nutrients, creating a symphony of nutrition that supports overall health and vitality.

1. Embrace a Variety of Protein Sources:
   - Vary your sources of protein to guarantee a wide range of nutrients. Incorporate lean meats, poultry, fish, plant-based proteins, legumes, and dairy products to receive a comprehensive array of amino acids and micronutrients.

2. Balance Macronutrients:
   - Maintain a balance between proteins, carbohydrates, and fats. Each macronutrient plays a unique role in supporting energy levels, hormone production, and overall cellular function. A balanced approach ensures your body receives a full spectrum of nutrients.

3. Opt for Whole Foods:
   - Choose whole, minimally processed foods to maximize nutrient density. Whole grains, fruits, vegetables, and unprocessed protein sources provide a wealth of vitamins, minerals, and fiber in addition to protein.

4. Mindful Portion Control:

- Practice portion control to prevent overconsumption of any specific nutrient. Be aware of serving sizes and adjust portions based on your individual nutritional needs, activity level, and health goals.

5. Include Healthy Fats:
  - Include foods high in healthy fats in your meals, such as olive oil, avocados, almonds, and seeds. Healthy fats contribute to satiety, support nutrient absorption, and play a crucial role in hormone regulation.

6. Prioritize Fiber-Rich Foods:
  - Integrate fiber-rich foods, including fruits, vegetables, whole grains, and legumes, into your diet. Fiber supports digestive health, promotes a feeling of fullness, and helps regulate blood sugar levels.

7. Stay Hydrated:
  - Adequate hydration is key to supporting overall health and optimizing nutrient absorption. Water is required for digestion, circulation, and nutrition movement throughout the body.

8. Consider Micronutrient Needs:
  - Pay attention to your micronutrient needs, including vitamins and minerals. Ensure your diet includes a variety of colorful fruits and vegetables to provide a spectrum of micronutrients that contribute to overall well-being.

9. Tailor Nutrition to Your Goals:
   - Consider your individual health and fitness goals when balancing nutrients. Whether you're focused on muscle building, weight management, or overall wellness, tailor your nutrition to align with your specific objectives.

10. Consult with a Nutrition Professional:
   - For personalized guidance, consult with a registered dietitian or nutrition professional. They can provide tailored advice based on your unique dietary preferences, health status, and lifestyle.

Balancing protein intake with other nutrients is a holistic approach to nutrition, ensuring that your body receives the diverse array of substances it needs to function optimally. By viewing your diet as a symphony of nutrients, you create a foundation for sustained energy, vitality, and long-term well-being.

CONCLUSION

Congratulations on embarking on a journey to embrace a high-protein lifestyle! This cookbook is not just a collection of recipes but a guide to transforming your daily meals into nourishing, protein-packed delights. As you've explored the diverse range of recipes and nutritional insights, I hope you've gained valuable knowledge and inspiration for creating meals that align with your health and fitness goals.

Remember, a high-protein lifestyle is about more than just the numbers on a nutrition label—it's a holistic approach to well-being. From understanding the role of protein in your diet to mastering meal prep and portion control, you've equipped yourself with tools to make informed and health-conscious choices.

Whether you're a seasoned chef or just starting in the kitchen, the recipes provided are designed to be both delicious and accessible. From energizing breakfasts to satisfying dinners and protein-packed snacks, this cookbook offers a variety of options to suit every palate.

As you savor the flavors of these recipes, pay attention to how your body responds. Listen to its cues, stay mindful of your nutritional needs, and enjoy the journey of discovering a balanced and sustainable approach to nutrition. Feel free to experiment, modify recipes to suit your taste, and make this high-protein lifestyle uniquely yours.

Thank you for choosing this cookbook as your companion on your quest for a healthier and protein-enriched life. May your culinary adventures be both fulfilling and nourishing. Here's to your well-being and the joy of savoring every bite on your high-protein journey!

Happy Cooking and Healthy Living!

CELEBRATING YOUR HEALTH AND WELLNESS JOURNEY

In the journey of health and wellness, celebrating your progress is as vital as the steps you take. "Celebrate Your Health and Wellness Journey" is an invitation to recognize, honor, and revel in the strides you've made towards a healthier, more vibrant you.

1. Reflect on Milestones:
  - Take a moment to reflect on the milestones you've achieved. Whether it's adopting a new fitness routine, making mindful food choices, or prioritizing self-care, each accomplishment deserves acknowledgment.

2. Nourish Your Body with Gratitude:

- Cultivate gratitude for your body and its incredible capabilities. Recognize the strength, resilience, and vitality that your wellness journey has brought forth. Nourishing your body becomes a celebration of the incredible vessel it is.

3. Embrace Mindful Eating Habits:
   - Celebrate the shift towards mindful eating. By savoring each bite with awareness, you not only enhance the pleasure of meals but also foster a positive relationship with food, supporting your overall well-being.

4. Cherish Balanced Choices:
   - Acknowledge the beauty of balanced choices. Whether it's incorporating more nutrient-dense foods, finding joy in regular physical activity, or practicing mindfulness, these choices contribute to a holistic approach to health.

5. Revel in Self-Care Rituals:
   - Identify and relish the self-care rituals that have become a cornerstone of your routine. Whether it's a calming evening walk, moments of meditation, or a cherished skincare routine, these rituals are a testament to your commitment to holistic well-being.

6. Explore Culinary Adventures:
   - Celebrate the joy of exploring new culinary horizons. Every wholesome meal, balanced snack, and nourishing recipe is a triumph on your health

journey. Allow the kitchen to be a canvas for creativity and self-expression.

7. Connect with Your Body:
   - Foster a deeper connection with your body. Celebrate its uniqueness, listen to its signals, and honor its needs. Your body is on a remarkable journey of its own, and embracing this connection is an integral part of your wellness celebration.

8. Share Your Achievements:
   - Don't hesitate to share your achievements with others. Whether it's with friends, family, or a supportive community, sharing your successes not only amplifies the joy but also inspires and motivates those around you.

9. Set New Intentions:
   - Celebrate by setting new intentions. Your wellness journey is ever-evolving, and each celebration is an opportunity to set new goals, aspirations, and intentions for continued growth and well-being.

10. Revel in the Present Moment:
   - Finally, celebrate by reveling in the present moment. Your health and wellness journey is a continuous process, and each moment is an opportunity to appreciate the gift of well-being. Allow yourself to bask in the gratitude of the here and now.

"Celebrate Your Health and Wellness Journey" is not just a phrase; it's an ethos that encourages you to acknowledge, embrace, and celebrate every facet of your journey towards a healthier, more fulfilled life. It's a reminder that self-love and self-celebration are integral components of the ongoing adventure towards well-being.

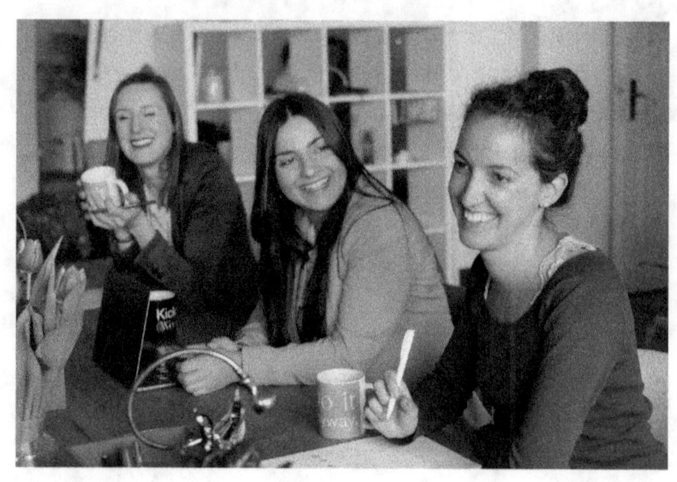